PSYCHEDELIC
MEDICINE

"Imagine that you could ask almost every noteworthy psychedelic researcher not only to discuss their work in depth outside of the jargon of heavy journal descriptions but also to discuss the implications of their work and where it will be going in the future. Imagine an interviewer that knows the research backward and forward and presses each person to think in new directions. It's all there in *Psychedelic Medicine*. I have been hoping for some years that there would be a book that I could point to that includes almost everything that's going on. This is as close as we're likely going to get. I'm in the book as well which is why I can attest to Miller's knowledgeable and invaluable questioning."

JAMES FADIMAN, PhD, MICRODOSE RESEARCHER AND
AUTHOR OF THE PSYCHEDELIC EXPLORER'S GUIDE: SAFE,
THERAPEUTIC, AND SPIRITUAL JOURNEYS

"We love Dr. Richard Miller's perceptive, up-close-and-personal interviews with the courageous pioneers of the psychedelic renaissance. *Psychedelic Medicine* is a treasure trove of insights into psychedelic-assisted psychotherapy's well-documented ability to facilitate lasting healing and life-changing mystical experience."

JERRY AND JULIE BROWN, COAUTHORS OF
THE PSYCHEDELIC GOSPELS: THE SECRET HISTORY
OF HALLUCINOGENS IN CHRISTIANITY

"Lively, in-depth, and insightful interviews with both pioneering and contemporary members of the psychedelic research community. An excellent introduction to many of the themes and figures involved in the recent resurgence of clinical studies with these drugs."

RICK STRASSMAN, MD,
AUTHOR OF *DMT: THE SPIRIT MOLECULE*
AND *DMT AND THE SOUL OF PROPHECY*

"Fascinating conversations between a veteran explorer of altered states of consciousness and many of the leading lights in a new wave of research into psychedelic-assisted therapy. Brings together the science and spirituality of the entheogenic revival."

DON LATTIN, AUTHOR OF *CHANGING OUR MINDS:
PSYCHEDELIC SACRAMENTS AND THE NEW PSYCHOTHERAPY*

"An amazing and inspiring read. Dr. Miller has cultivated provocative conversations with luminaries in the field of psychedelic research as well as some solid criticism of modern psychiatry."

JULIE HOLLAND, MD, EDITOR OF *THE POT BOOK*
AND *ECSTASY: THE COMPLETE GUIDE*
AND AUTHOR OF *MOODY BITCHES* AND
WEEKENDS AT BELLEVUE

PSYCHEDELIC
MEDICINE

The Healing Powers of LSD, MDMA, Psilocybin, and Ayahuasca

Dr. Richard Louis Miller

Park Street Press
Rochester, Vermont • Toronto, Canada

Park Street Press
One Park Street
Rochester, Vermont 05767
www.ParkStPress.com

SUSTAINABLE FORESTRY INITIATIVE — Certified Sourcing — www.sfiprogram.org — SFI-00854

Text stock is SFI certified

Park Street Press is a division of Inner Traditions International

Library of Congress Cataloging-in-Publication Data

Names: Miller, Richard Louis, author.
Title: Psychedelic medicine : the healing powers of LSD, MDMA, Psilocybin, and Ayahuasca / Dr. Richard Louis Miller.
Description: Rochester, Vermont : Park Street Press, [2017] | Includes bibliographical references and index.
Identifiers: LCCN 2017007943 (print) | LCCN 2017009109 (e-book) | ISBN 9781620556979 (paperback) | ISBN 9781620556986 (e-book)
Subjects: LCSH: Hallucinogenic drugs—Therapeutic use. | Psychotherapy. | BISAC: HEALTH & FITNESS / Alternative Therapies. | SOCIAL SCIENCE / Popular Culture.
Classification: LCC RM324.8 M55 2017 (print) | LCC RM324.8 (e-book) | DDC 615.7/883—dc23
LC record available at https://lccn.loc.gov/2017007943

Printed and bound in the United States by Lake Book Manufacturing, Inc. The text stock is SFI certified. The Sustainable Forestry Initiative® program promotes sustainable forest management.

10 9 8 7 6 5

Text design by Priscilla H. Baker and layout by Virginia Scott Bowman
This book was typeset in Garamond Premier Pro with Antonio and Gill Sans used as display typeface

To send correspondence to the author of this book, mail a first-class letter to the author c/o Inner Traditions • Bear & Company, One Park Street, Rochester, VT 05767, and we will forward the communication, or contact the author directly at **www.mindbodyhealthpolitics.org**.

Contents

About the Author

Dr. Richard Louis Miller is an American clinical psychologist, owner of Wilbur Hot Springs Sanctuary for the Self, and radio broadcaster who hosts *Mind, Body, Health & Politics,* which airs on National Public Radio affiliate KZYX FM in Mendocino County, California.

Dr. Miller was the founder and chief clinician of the nationally acclaimed and highly successful Cokenders Alcohol and Drug Program. This pioneering program viewed chemical dependence as an opportunity to enter the world of health through group, individual, and family therapy, along with mindful awareness training, yoga, aerobic exercise, nutrition education, art therapy, breath training, and right livelihood.

During his long career Dr. Miller was on the faculties of the University of Michigan and Stanford University; served as division president of Parkside Medical Services Corporation, the country's largest provider of chemical dependence treatment; was consultant to the Haight Ashbury Free Medical Clinic and the New Hampshire Division of Alcoholism; and gave testimony before the California Assembly and the President's Commission on Mental Health. He is presently in private practice in Fort Bragg and Wilbur Springs, California, where he lives with his wife, Jolee; two Rhodesian ridgebacks, Abigail and Franklin; one Borzoi, Sasha; one Angus steer, Brownie CowSanova; five goats; three chickens; two ducks; and seven cats.

What's Happening in America?

This book offers the reader interviews with leading scientists in America who are investigating the effects on humans of the psychedelic medicines LSD, MDMA, psilocybin, and ayahuasca. *Psychedelic Medicine* is an expression of fifty years of my professional and personal interest in the medicinal and transformational benefits of psychedelics substances.

I received my first license to practice clinical psychology in 1966 while teaching psychology at the University of Michigan in Ann Arbor. One evening a colleague invited me to his home where he offered me the opportunity to experience DMT (dimethyltriptamine). I took one puff of the normal appearing cigarette, immediately closed my eyes, lay back, and explored the very deepest core of my consciousness and the very borders of the universe.

I had a clear sense that within the infinite universes I was smaller than what I see while using an electron microscope. I experienced being and nothingness. The experience lasted about twelve minutes. I sat up and asked for another puff. Once again I embarked on inner-space travel. I became a dematerialized inner-space traveler transcending time. I soared through the universe in search of the Source. I had a clear sense that I was a part of, an expression of, the whole of it all. My journey had begun.

I began to research what science had to say about these medicines, and why the United States government declared them non grata to an extent that profoundly obstructed scientific research into them.

In the years following I had the good fortune to participate in experimental sessions with LSD, MDMA, mescaline, psilocybin, ketamine, and marijuana. These introspective experiences were exciting, educational, enhancing, frightening, spiritual, captivating, and healing.

Looking back at the past half century, and reading what the scientists in this book have brought us, it is abundantly clear that the American public has been denied access to medicines having potential to change the course of human history. For those of us who share the belief that within us all is innate wisdom, accessing the Deep Within is our life path. Many avenues to the Deep Within have been explored, including meditation, mindfulness, yoga, stimulus isolation tanks, anechoic chambers, monastic living, ingesting organic matter from the ground, and ingesting synthetic matter from laboratories.

America's leading scientists in psychedelic research, interviewed in this book, bring data revealing that certain psychedelic medicines, administered by proper protocols, informed by research and clearly described, offer altered states of consciousness facilitating brilliant creativity and psychophysical healing. Witness the findings of deep healing led by Roland Griffiths at Johns Hopkins, Charles Grob at UCLA, Dave Nichols at Indiana University, and Michael Mithofer of MAPS. Witness also the creativity of astrophysicist Carl Sagan, Apple founder Steve Jobs, physicist Richard Feynman, DNA scientist Francis Crick, and neuroscientist John Lilly, all of whom utilized psychedelics in their professional work and discoveries.

Imagine taking a medicine that alters your mind and facilitates the generation of new thoughts and new ways of looking at the world.

Imagine taking a medicine that facilitates solving problems of life, be they personal or professional.

Imagine taking a medicine for the purpose of spiritual prophylaxis, the cleansing of the spirit that has been clogged up by life.

When we expand our consciousness we liberate ourselves from the slavery that is inherent in all cultural and institutional systems. The slavery derives from repetition of daily life until the behavior becomes institutionalized, thereby creating culture. Rigidified, institutionalized culture is the ultimate peer pressure, which stifles, dominates, and controls both creativity and consciousness expansion.

Once a person ingests a psychedelic medicine and experiences the Deep Within and expanded consciousness, there is no going back to narrow consciousness and constricted thinking. What has been seen cannot be unseen. Once we experience alternate realities we can never again say this is the only one reality. When we experience ourselves as electrochemical beings of light, as molecules stuck together taking material form, our lives take on new meaning.

Psychedelic medicine can facilitate our using the power of the mind to change our very genetic structure. We can change the slings and arrows of outrageous genetic misfortune into a Cupid's bow of a sculpted self.

A Call for Transparency
April 3, 2012

Recently I was walking down a country road over at Wilbur Hot Springs in Colusa County, California, and I met a Danish couple— about twenty-five, twenty-six years old—and we began chatting. At one point they looked at me with the most innocent of eyes and said, "What is happening to your country?"

I looked around, and I said, "What?"

They said, "What has happened to your country? We know that

something bad is happening to your country, but we don't understand it. Can you tell us about it?"

The world seems to know that something has happened, and is happening, to our country. I'm sure you are aware of it. Or are you? It's not an easy thing to grasp. Sometimes, when we see things happening to a country, or to our county or city, we might ask ourselves: Is this just me or am I the victim of some conspiratorial thinking? Is it just me and my little group of friends or is this actually happening? Well, it is actually happening. In this book, I'm going to expose part of what is happening—namely the long-term suppression of one kind of scientific information. Suppression of information is symptomatic.

Perhaps some of you who regularly listen to my radio program have asked yourselves why I'm doing this lengthy series on psychedelic medicines. My radio program is about mind, body, health, and politics. It's about bringing you what I consider to be truth—meaning what's really happening out there. What's going on in the world of mind, body, health, and politics that the public is not being told about? That's what I mean by truth—getting it all out there and being transparent. I believe in transparency. I believe we, the citizens, have a right to know everything—and I mean everything. I think secrets cause problems. They cause division among human beings, whereas transparency brings us together. We all want to be in the know. We don't want to feel that we're being excluded.

Information is power, and having more information can lead to having power over others, or having power to share with others. There has been suppression of information in our country for a long time. Our original Constitution was a landmark in the history of the world, but there's a lot of work that needs to be done on it. And what's new about that? Thomas Jefferson told us over two hundred years ago that the Constitution should be rewritten every twenty years, for every new generation, because otherwise it gets out of date. I'm not claiming to be saying anything new.

The area of psychedelic medicine has been suppressed from the public for so long and for so many reasons that we're out of reasons. There are no *good* reasons for suppressing university research on medicine. There are just *reasons*. This lack of information is hurting people, because scientists are telling us that there is healing that can be achieved through the use of these medicines, and people are being denied this healing. At least if the information about the medicines were allowed to the public they would be able to make their own decisions. I ask myself: Why would the government suppress research? This is what I intend to explore.

What Determines Policy: Science or Ideology?

Former president Barack Obama told CNN medical correspondent Sanjay Gupta, MD, that our government's health policy regarding marijuana should be directed by science and not ideology. This admonition by our learned former president is contrary to the prevailing reality of how our government functions and how laws are made.

Case in point: In 1930 Secretary of the Treasury Andrew Mellon (of the Mellon banking family) appointed his relative Harry J. Anslinger to be commissioner of the Federal Bureau of Narcotics. Mr. Anslinger clearly favored religion and ideology over science. His ideology included a manic, obsessive hatred of people of color. As a result, for the past eighty-seven years the American people—and the world—have suffered from Mr. Anslinger's racist ideology. Lives have been lost, families shattered, cities damaged, and entire governments such as Mexico's have been threatened by Mr. Harry Anslinger's successful creation of laws that enforced his ideology while ignoring science.

Anslinger, along with others, prosecuted the Chinese for using opium, the Mexicans for marijuana, and blacks for cocaine. Disinformation was spread that these minority people of color were using the drugs to seduce white women, and the public roared. By using the mass media as his forum (receiving much support from yellow journalism publisher William Randolph Hearst), Anslinger propelled the antimarijuana sentiment from state level to a national, and then international, movement. He used what he called his Gore Files—a collection of quotes from police reports—to graphically depict offenses caused by drug users.

By representing the United States before the United Nations, Harry Anslinger made certain substances illegal on a worldwide scale. Alcohol prohibition in the United States lasted thirteen years, during which time two issues became obvious. First, the American people were not going to be legislated out of drinking alcohol. Second, making alcohol illegal spawned a criminal enterprise that we call the mafia, whose gross revenue approached the nation's entire (previously legal) alcoholic beverage industry. It's hard to wrap your consciousness around that! Take every business in the United States that is involved with alcohol, from the production to the distribution to the sales—every bit of it: hard spirits, beer, and wine—and that is the amount of business that we gave to the criminal enterprise. It might not be a stretch to say that Harry Anslinger created the largest, most successful criminal enterprise the world has ever known. When Harry Anslinger waged a war on alcohol, and Richard Nixon and Ronald Reagan subsequently declared a war on drugs, they were in fact declaring a war on people—mostly people of color. Eighty-seven years after Mr. Anslinger's federal appointment and his creation of the marijuana tax laws of 1937, our jails are burdened with an ocean of people of color whose only crime was an act of ingesting a vegetable, marijuana, that comes from the ground.

While people of color make up about 30 percent of the United States' population, they account for 60 percent of those imprisoned. The incarceration rates in America disproportionately impact men of color: 1 in every 15 African American men and 1 in every 36 Hispanic men are incarcerated in comparison to 1 in every 106 white men.

In recent decades, people around the United States have responded to this war against people by attempting to bring science into this ideological war. Pioneering groups such as the Drug Policy Alliance,

National Organization to Reform Marijuana Law (NORML), the Multidisciplinary Association for Psychedelic Studies (MAPS), and the Marijuana Policy Project (MPP) advance the cause of overturning drug laws driven by ideology.

When our forty-fourth American president, Barack Obama, called for the acceptance of science over ideology, we thought we saw the end of Harry Anslinger's eighty-five-year rule. We were mistaken.

A Call to Freedom

Following Anslinger's lead, most governments around the world have taken a strong position against the cause of personal freedom. By making certain substances illegal, even in the laboratory of science, they have curtailed basic rights and constitutional rights.

However, in recent years, the United States government has allowed a very limited amount of research into psychoactive substances. It is this political breakthrough that fueled many of the interviews provided in this book, which have been transcribed from my radio program *Mind, Body, Health & Politics*. My program is known for its wide-ranging discussions on political issues and health. The show's format includes guest interviews, guest speakers, and listener call-ins, offering a forum and soundboard for listeners to interact with the hosts and their guests.

Within this platform, I have had the opportunity to interview leading scientists in the field of psychedelic research. Each of the scientists interviewed in this book has made monumental contributions to understanding human consciousness. Taken together, including the political climate in which they conducted their research, their work makes them heroic figures.

On the very frontiers of inner-space travel, these scientists have significantly impacted the philosophical and political cause of freedom. Freedom to explore oneself and to express one's findings to anyone interested is one of the great causes of humanity.

The scientists interviewed in this book have dedicated their lives to doing their research within the law and presenting their findings to the world. It is reasonable to believe they risked their reputations, their convenience, and perhaps their lives.

It has been my great honor to interview each of them, and it is with much pleasure that I offer you their book.

ONE

LSD

A Powerful Tool

Substance: LSD-25 (lysergic acid diethylamide), also known as acid
and LSD
Schedule: I*

A Brief History of LSD

LSD—lysergic acid diethylamide—was first synthesized on November 16, 1938, by Swiss chemist Albert Hofmann at Sandoz Laboratories in Basel, Switzerland, as part of a large research program searching for medically useful ergot-alkaloid derivatives. LSD's psychedelic properties were discovered five years later, when Hofmann himself accidentally ingested an unknown quantity of the chemical.

The first *intentional* ingestion of LSD occurred some years later in 1943, when Hofmann himself ingested 250 micrograms—yes, micrograms.[†] He said this would be a threshold dose based on the dosages of other ergot alkaloids. Well, Hofmann found the effects to be

---

*No recognized medical use and high potential for abuse.
[†]1/1,000,000 of a gram.

much stronger than he anticipated. After ingesting the LSD, Hofmann got on his bicycle to go home. This came to be known as one of the most famous bike rides in all of history.

Sandoz Laboratories introduced LSD as a psychiatric drug in 1947. Then, beginning in the 1950s, the United States Central Intelligence Agency began a research program code-named Project MKUltra. Experiments included administering LSD to CIA employees, military personnel, doctors, other government agents, prostitutes, mentally ill patients, and members of the general public. Some believe—in fact, *many* believe—they usually studied subjects' reactions without the subjects' knowledge.

The project was revealed in the U.S. Congressional Rockefeller Commission Report (on CIA activities in the United States) in 1975. In 1963, Sandoz's patents expired. The same year, in 1963, the U.S. Food and Drug Administration classified LSD as an Investigational New Drug, which meant there were new restrictions on medical and scientific use. Several figures, including Aldous Huxley, Timothy Leary, and others, began to advocate the consumption of LSD, and it became central to the counterculture of the 1960s. Then, on October 24, 1968, possession of LSD was made illegal in the United States.

The last FDA-approved study of LSD in patients ended in 1980, while a study with healthy volunteers was made in the late '80s. For the most part, research into LSD has been suppressed in this country. Why is that? By classifying LSD as a Schedule I substance, the Drug Enforcement Agency (DEA) holds that LSD meets the following three criteria:

1) It is deemed to have a high potential for abuse.
2) It has no legitimate medical use and treatment.
3) There is a lack of accepted safety for its use under medical supervision.

Leading the Way
Four Pioneering Researchers on LSD

When it comes to LSD, there are four prominent scientists we will be talking with: David Nichols, PhD, an American pharmacologist and medicinal chemist; Amanda Feilding, Countess of Wemyss and March, an English artist, scientist, and drug-policy reformer; Stanislav Grof, MD, PhD, a Czech psychiatrist, one of the founders of the field of transpersonal psychology and a researcher into the use of nonordinary states of consciousness; and James Fadiman, PhD, an American psychologist, author, researcher, and lecturer in psychedelic studies.

A Seminar for
the Like-minded

In the mid-1980s, the Esalen Institute held a special—by invitation only—seminar, inviting the very few scientists in the United States who were allowed by the U.S. government to conduct research on psychedelic medicines.

It was at this seminar that I first met Dave Nichols, PhD, a professor of medicinal chemistry and molecular pharmacology at Purdue University. Nichols is our country's, if not the world's, leading scientist on the subject of LSD. Mild-mannered and straightforward, with no agenda other than pure science, he was the perfect person to conduct research on a topic that garnered so much controversy. Being one of the only—if not the only—scientists allowed to research LSD, a great deal of weight has been on Nichols's shoulders. Here, we shall find out some of what he has to report.

The Biochemistry of Changes in Consciousness

David Nichols, PhD

November 15, 2011

DAVID NICHOLS, PHD, holds the Robert C. and Charlotte P. Anderson distinguished chair in pharmacology at Purdue University College of Pharmacy. He is also a distinguished professor of medicinal chemistry and molecular pharmacology and is an adjunct professor of pharmacology and toxicology at the Indiana University School of Medicine. Dave has published nearly three hundred scientific articles and is recognized as one of the world's foremost authorities on the chemistry and pharmacology of psychedelics.

Learning from the Past, Working in the Present

Early Research Cut Short by DEA Scheduling

Dr. Richard Louis Miller (RLM): Welcome to *Mind, Body, Health & Politics,* Dave.

David Nichols, PhD (DN): Good morning.

RLM: The DEA holds that LSD meets the criteria for Schedule I substances, that is, it is deemed to have a high potential for abuse, has no legitimate medical use and treatment, and there is a lack of accepted safety for its use under medical supervision. What does your research have to say?

DN: To begin with, the DEA's definition of high potential for abuse really means that people will take it without a prescription. It doesn't necessarily mean that it has the possibility of getting people addicted. On the safety issue, LSD has never killed anyone directly from overdose. It's a fairly benign substance from a physiological point of view. Now, that doesn't mean that it can't lead to psychological problems, but from a physiological point of view it's pretty safe. Also, lack of medical uses were really never documented. The research was nipped in the bud.

LSD's Mark on the Field of Behavioral Psychology

DN: There was a lot of enthusiasm when LSD sprang on the scene in the early 1950s. In fact, it catalyzed a lot of neuroscience research. The selective serotonin reuptake inhibitors [SSRIs] we use now for treating depression probably wouldn't have arrived as quickly as they did if LSD hadn't been discovered. Because of the profound effects of LSD on the human psyche, it really was the first point at which neuroscientists realized that there was a connection between brain chemistry and behavior. Prior to that time, if a child became schizophrenic, they would blame the parents or the mother, figuring the parents failed or that breastfeeding had failed.

There was no recognition that brain chemistry had anything to do with behavior. That seems kind of amazing today, but that actually was the situation. It was only within a few years of the discovery of LSD that *serotonin was discovered in the brain.* Looking at those two structures, researchers realized LSD actually has the same kind of chemical template as serotonin, and serotonin was in the brain, and LSD produces these dramatic behavioral changes—so they realized maybe there is some relationship between brain serotonin and behavior.

Early LSD Research:
A Scattershot Approach with Promising Prospects

DN: With all of the enthusiasm and excitement, they tried LSD in almost any imaginable condition: for autism . . . alcoholism . . . sexual dysfunction. You name it, they tried it—to see what it could do. It was usually given by poorly trained therapists, or lay therapists, or self-proclaimed therapists, because you could get the drug easily.

There were thousands of papers published on the uses of LSD, but they weren't done to rigorous standards. So we don't really know what can be done. There certainly were tantalizing hints that LSD might be useful in treating alcoholism or substance abuse. One of the best-documented uses was for treating anxiety and depression in terminal cancer patients. Between 60 and 70 percent had alleviation of symptoms and, in some cases, a reduction in need for pain medication. Under proper medical supervision, the safety of LSD was not really an issue. When used in a proper and appropriate medical context, the incidence of adverse effects is very small.

How University Research Is Suppressed

Lack of Funding and Champions for the Cause

RLM: Why is the research still so limited among serious university researchers like yourself?

DN: Research is driven by funding mechanisms. For almost thirty years, I was funded by the National Institute on Drug Abuse [NIDA] to study hallucinogens, or psychedelics. My research is fundamentally focused on how they work in the brain. How do they produce their effects? When there is widespread use in the population, NIDA says we should throw some money at it. So for cocaine, MDMA, and new synthetic cannabinoids like "Spice," they say, "We need to look at that." So they put money there. People were not using hallucinogens to that great of an extent. That's part of it. Also, government agencies are driven by in-house programs that study marijuana, cocaine, methamphetamine, and so forth—all the substances that are serious problems in their view—so that's where they put the money. Hallucinogens are not really something they're that concerned with.

Since these substances became controlled, and especially Schedule I, you have to receive a special license to study them. You have to say exactly how you're going to use LSD, how much you're going to use, and how long you're going to use it. That all has to be approved by the DEA, and I believe they now even include the FDA in requiring approval. The approval process can take anywhere from six months to two years, and then you have to have a secure place to store the substance—even if it's a relatively small amount. Suppose you ordered five milligrams of LSD, which wouldn't be a huge amount. The DEA's concern is that you would still need the same kind of storage safeguards and record keeping you would need if you had much larger amounts. Scientists know this is a hassle, and they don't want to have to do this. I have to get a special registration and I have to pay a fee. With respect to clinical research, that's an order of magnitude—more regulation than animal or test-tube research.

RLM: So a person needs a great deal of inherent interest to want to go through the hassle and impediments of getting the protocols accepted?

DN: Basically, you need personal motivation or reasons to devote yourself to this kind of activity. For example, it has taken a few years to get approval for the recent studies with psilocybin. You also need approval by the institutional review board.

There are maybe half a dozen people in the world who really believe that these things have some value and have a sort of personal commitment to making it happen. But you don't see a large-scale movement to study these substances, in contrast to something like cancer or HIV/AIDS. Everyone is aware that cancer is a big problem. A young researcher might have had somebody in her family who had cancer, so she will go into cancer research. Or maybe someone had an acquaintance die of HIV/AIDS. You don't have the feeling in the population that psychedelics are really an important field. It takes a personal commitment by a few people, whom I would call visionary, to look at this and say, "There is something there that's valuable, and we need to pick through it, find little nuggets, find out what they are, and bring them out for medicine."

Psychedelics: A "Career Killer"

RLM: When I was a young graduate student, there were some topics of research we were told were almost career killers. One of them was hypnosis, for example. I remember talking to Ernest Hilgard of Stanford University, a behaviorist who did years of rat research until he eventually became a full professor at Stanford, after which he began doing research into hypnosis. Hilgard said to me directly, "I made my career in rats so that I could finally do the hypnosis research. I knew if I went into hypnosis first, I'd never get anywhere."

DN: Studying psychedelics would be another career killer for most people.

RLM: You're saying there's about a half dozen around the country . . . that's like Roland Griffiths at Johns Hopkins doing the psilocybin research that's been getting some press . . . Charles Grob down at Harbor-UCLA Medical . . .

DN: Right, also Steve Ross. We have another fellow, Michael Bogenschutz, at University of New Mexico that is now looking at psilocybin in treatment of alcoholism. And then Franz Vollenweider in Zurich, Switzerland, has a laboratory where he's doing a lot of basic clinical science research. All of these people are actually involved in the Heffter Research Institute, which I founded in 1993 to carry out legitimate research with these substances.

The Biggest Job Requirement for a Psychedelic Pharmacologist: Curiosity

DN: In 1970 we had the Controlled Substances Act, and soon these things all became illegal. I had studied the chemistry of these substances as a graduate student from 1969 to 1973, and I was looking forward to doing some pharmacological work and understanding how they worked. In fact, I did a postdoctoral fellowship in pharmacology in the College of Medicine at Iowa, and then I finished up, and they were illegal.

RLM: What piqued your interest to continue?

DN: I say to people, "Think of the things that can change your life, okay? You fall in love, get married, have a child . . . maybe a parent dies, a sibling dies, or child dies . . . or you get divorced . . . or you take a dose of LSD . . ." And suddenly people are caught off guard, and they look at you and say, "LSD?"

I say, "Yes. How is it possible that if you ingest a tiny amount of this substance, it will diffuse into your brain, stay for three or four hours, and diffuse back out, such that some people say they never see the world in the same way again? Some people are permanently changed for good or for bad, depending. How is it possible that a molecule can do that?"

I had been interested in philosophy—Who are we? How did we get here? What is man?—not real well-formed ideas. But it occurred to me . . . a drug that could do this must be interacting in a very fundamental place in the brain, a place that is important to determining who we are, how we perceive the world around us, and how we interact.

Unlocking the Secrets of Neuroscience

DN: When I started in the medicinal chemistry department, I developed what is called structure-activity series. You make a series of molecules, and you look at how active they are, and then you try to figure out why one was more active than the other. To use a crude analogy: You have a lock, and you don't know what the proper key is, so you keep making keys and find out that in the first position it will push one of the tumblers up. You keep making more keys until you know whether or not a particular part of the key would activate one of the tumblers in the lock. Eventually you get a key that opens the lock. In medicinal chemistry, you make lots of related molecules with similar structures and then you do some kind of a biological assay [determination of the potency or quality of each molecule's effect] and determine how potent they are with respect to each other. You look at the most potent and least potent, and you ask what they have in common and how they differ. This was an indirect way for me to probe, "Where is the site in the brain where they bind? What is the site 'looking for' when it binds these substances?"

RLM: Were you yourself taking LSD at the time during graduate school?

DN: No. Maybe I would have made more discoveries if I had been. Basically I was figuring out how to make these synthetic compounds. It was clear that a lot of these compounds, called substituted amphetamines [related to mescaline], had optical isomers, meaning they were sort of two forms. Nobody had found a good way to make those two forms, and as a graduate student, I found a way that we subsequently patented. I was making tools and finding molecules that other people could use in their models to do the assays. I really didn't do much in the way of biological assays until my postdoctoral work.

The Mystery of a Mind-Changing Molecule

RLM: One dose of LSD can create life change. That is what you're talking about, and that is what many of us know. Why?

DN: I can't give you the answer to that question at this point.

RLM: Still under investigation?

DN: Yes. LSD is unique among all of these compounds. You have mescaline and there are a whole series of derivatives that have names like DOB, DOI, 2C-I, and 2C-B. None of them really have the profundity of effect that you see with LSD.

We're trying to figure out what LSD does that makes it different from these others, and we haven't really discovered what it is. We think part of the secret is that LSD interacts with a dozen or so receptors, whereas if you look at something like mescaline or psilocybin, they really only interact powerfully with a couple of brain receptors. But we've been doing studies looking at the actual receptor itself that these drugs bind to, mutating and changing the amino acids, and looking at how these drugs bind. LSD has this one feature—the *diethylamide* part of lysergic acid diethylamide—that seems to interact with this flap at the top of the receptor. We've made about twenty-five different derivatives where we've made the *diethyls* into rings—big rings, small rings, and all kinds of things. When we make a change like that the molecule invariably loses about 90 percent of its activity in the models we used. So there is something going on with that diethylamide. We think that the receptor folds over and interacts in way that produces a change in the receptor that we haven't quantified yet. It's a very complex problem, though.

A Serotonergic Clue

DN: All of the psychedelics also interact or activate the serotonin 5-HT_{2A} receptor.

RLM: Why is serotonin so important, and why does it get so much press?

DN: Serotonin is a very ancient and foundational neurotransmitter. There are three kinds of what we call monoamine neurotransmitters in the brain: dopamine, norepinephrine, and serotonin. All of these transmitters are produced by neurons that come from groups of cell bodies at the top of the brain stem, or in the lower midbrain—right where the spinal cord enters the brain. The raphe nuclei are neurons that make serotonin and send their projections to all parts of the brain.

There are fifteen different types of receptors known for serotonin—far more than for dopamine and norepinephrine. If you build a phylogenetic tree, you find that serotonin goes way back into evolutionary history, occurring in paramecia and simple insects. It was employed early on in evolution for a variety of things—including brain development and all kinds of systems development. In humans, we know that serotonin neurons project into virtually all parts of the cortex and higher areas of the brain. They're involved in emotions—anger, rage, hunger, sex drive, cognition, depression, mood, and more.

LSD Modulates Information the Brain Counts as Relevant

RLM: So it is a major information transmitter?

DN: Well, dopamine, serotonin, and norepinephrine are really *modulators* of other systems. The real hardwiring in the brain uses fast transmitters, such as glutamate and gamma-aminobutyric acid [GABA], and to some extent acetylcholine. Serotonin, dopamine, and norepinephrine will modulate those systems—regulate them up and down. The hardware is driven by glutamate and GABA, and ion transport. Serotonin modulates those systems and makes them more reactive or less reactive. That's probably the best analogy I can give.

The most ancient, as far as I can tell, are the serotonin 2 receptors, which come in three variations: 2A, 2B, and 2C. It turns out that the serotonin 2A receptor is heavily expressed in a lot of the areas of the brain involved in cognition and higher cortical processing. It's also heavily expressed in the primary visual cortex, so with low doses of psychedelics you see a lot of visual illusions and distortions. People say the walls are melting, or they see moving patterns in carpets, and so forth.

RLM: What's happening when one seems to see the desk breathing, or the wall breathing—like a Dali painting, where the pieces seem to be melting? Are these illusions or distortions?

DN: The first place visual information goes is from the eyes into the primary visual cortex, and so it clearly is going to be corrupted at that level, but then it gets processed at higher centers, where you put it together to make sense out of it. All of that architecture is affected by LSD as well.

There are also serotonin 2A receptors in the area called the thalamus and in the reticular nucleus of the thalamus—a gateway center in the brain that decides what sensory information gets sent to the cortex for processing. Normally, in everyday life, you're not attending to every possible thing that's going on in your body or around you: the muscles that are maintaining your posture, the temperature in the room, or noise you've become accustomed to. Your brain shuts out the things that are not relevant sensory information.

There are serotonin 2A receptors in the part of the brain referred to as the searchlight of attention, the locus coeruleus, which is a novelty detector. So if something in your environment happens that is novel—if you turn around when you hear somebody slam the door in your studio—your locus coeruleus starts firing and calling your attention to it.

There are serotonin 1A receptors in the raphe nuclei themselves, which are the cell bodies that send out these serotonin projections to all parts of the brain, and they also fire at different rates, depending upon whether their serotonin 1A receptors are activated. LSD also activates serotonin 1A receptors.

RLM: So the serotonin that the public hears about—particularly with the advent of the SSRIs—it's not sending different messages, each having a direct effect. Rather, it is a modulator, or a governor, of the serotonin that is having an effect on these other neurotransmitters. So it is your serotonin governor that's being affected when serotonin is affected, is that correct?

DN: Yes, psychedelics activate serotonin 2A receptors, which are important in determining your level of awareness, your vigilance, your cognitive processing. These receptors are heavily expressed on neurons in the prefrontal cortex, where you make your executive decisions . . . where everything kind of comes together, and you create your own reality. Psychedelics change the firing frequency of those cells, so every place in the brain that is involved in cognition and consciousness is directly or indirectly affected when psychedelics stimulate these serotonin 2A receptors.

The Interplay of
Serotonin 2A and 2C Activation

DN: All of the psychedelics activate the 2A and 2C receptors about equally. In some cases they are even more effective at the 2C receptor than at the 2A receptor. The interesting thing is that activation of the 2A and 2C receptors produces opposite effects on brain chemistry. Activation of the 2A receptor enhances the formation and release of dopamine. Activation of the 2C receptor suppresses formation and release of dopamine. These two receptors in various parts of the brain actually oppose each other. All the studies have suggested that the key thing a psychedelic does is activate the serotonin 2A receptor, and they ignore what goes on at the 2C receptor because it doesn't seem to be a player. For a long time I wanted to try to find a way to develop a drug that would be specific and only activate the 2A receptor without activating the 2C receptor.

RLM: To increase the dopamine . . . and that's the connection with your Parkinson's research, I imagine?

DN: It goes beyond that. There are a whole host of functions where the two receptors just antagonize each other. So dopamine has one effect, but there are lots of others. We recently stumbled on a way to actually just activate 2A receptors. We're now making some compounds that are selective for serotonin 2A receptors, just to make them as tools for people to use to say, "Okay, now you've got a drug that only activates the serotonin 2A receptor." I've spent a lot of time with the Heffter Research Institute— although I'm not a clinician—dialoguing and trying to keep that fundraising going, and getting investigators interested in doing clinical research.

The Quantum Change in Consciousness

High-Dose Unpredictability

RLM: How do you connect the size of the psychological effect with the psychopharmacological effect that you've been describing for us?

DN: I believe there is actually a sort of quantum change in consciousness when people have these life-changing events. At lower doses, sensory information is all that's being altered by this drug—the curtains breathe, walls breathe, maybe you close your eyes and see colored patterns that move with the music—but at a certain point, and at some doses, it's unpredictable. In a lot of cases, all that external sensory change in your environment disappears, and you are projected into a novel environment of another place and time. It may have beings in it. It may not have beings. You may have a perception of a creator. There is something different that happens there that no one has been able to trap yet.

Roland Griffiths at Johns Hopkins found that something like 60 percent of people had what he called a "mystical transcendental experience" (see chapter 3). In all of the research with psychedelics, when they've seen a permanent, powerful change, it has generally occurred following one of these intense mystical transcendental experiences that is ineffable . . . indescribable. People believe in some cases that they have had a vision of paradise or that they have spoken with God, or Buddha, or whatever. Nobody understands what happens there, and I think there's fundamentally a difference that occurs—some kind of a quantum state in the brain that changes. No one knows exactly how or why that happens, but it has to be related to these 2A receptors.

RLM: What is the higher dose that occasions these experiences?

DN: It's rare to see that happen for the kinds of doses that are available on the street today—between 20 and 60 micrograms—although under the right circumstances it could. But in the '60s, when LSD was available on the street in tablets containing between 150 and 400 micrograms, most people who took a dose like that would have difficulty maintaining contact with the environment they were familiar with. But a high dose doesn't guarantee that, and a low dose doesn't preclude that.

Resetting Behavioral Subroutines

RLM: Do we know what size dose is best for psychotherapeutic use?

DN: It depends upon the kind of psychotherapy. There were two kinds of therapies: psycholytic and psychedelic. Psycholytic was where you would give a relatively low dose to the person and engage them in cognitive therapy—talk therapy, if you will.

Psychedelic therapy was where you really didn't do much except prepare the patient beforehand and give them a very large, overwhelming dose. The idea was that if you prepared them correctly, their own brain and mind would realize what the problem was and come to a solution.

A really interesting case was published back in the '70s about an individual that developed severe obsessive-compulsive disorder. He had to quit his job because he would have to wash his hands a dozen times and use four rolls of toilet paper every time he went to the bathroom. He was given LSD without any therapy at all—just put in the room and told to think about whatever—and there was a nurse and doctor available. The patient took LSD, virtually alone, about once a month for a year, and he completely recovered his normal personality, got his job back, and his friends and relatives said he was better than ever. There wasn't any therapy involved other than the LSD.

So the goal of psychedelic therapy is to produce a transcendental mystical state where you get a different perspective on things. Nobody can explain how it happens. I use the analogy of rebooting a computer. I believe we may accumulate what are called behavioral subroutines during life. These start to control the way you feel, the way you think, and so forth. We are not aware of them, because they're running in a subliminal way. Whatever this psychedelic effect is, it somehow reboots and inactivates some of these dysfunctional behaviors. I'm just speculating on the evidence.

RLM: A very interesting way of looking at it.

•••

Artist, Researcher, Reformer

Now, I want to move on to my second interviewee, researcher Amanda Feilding. I am very fortunate to be able to include her historic research on brain imaging and LSD in this book, because this cutting-edge information became available after the initial draft of this book was completed. I met Amanda's son, Cosmo, at the Mendocino International Film Festival where I sponsored and introduced a film he made, *The Sunshine Makers*. *The Sunshine Makers* is about the Brotherhood of Eternal Love, which at one time was one of the world's largest distributors of LSD. Subsequently I was introduced to Amanda by my good friend Nick Cozzi, PhD, a research medical pharmacologist at the University of Wisconsin. Amanda is a major force in England toward creating medicine policies based on science.

LSD Brain-Imaging Studies
Amanda Feilding
Excerpt from July 7, 2016

AMANDA FEILDING is an English artist, scientist, and drug-policy reformer. In 1998 Amanda founded the Beckley Foundation, a charitable trust that promotes a rational, evidence-based approach to global drug policy and initiates, designs, and carries out pioneering neuroscientific and clinical research into the effects of psychoactive substances on the brain and on cognition. She is dedicated to investigating novel treatment pathways for mental and physical conditions as well as developing new means to enhance creativity and well-being.

RLM: Today we've got an exciting interview with researcher Amanda Feilding. Welcome to *Mind, Body, Health & Politics,* Amanda.

Amanda Feilding (AF): Thank you.

RLM: My understanding is that you originally set up the Beckley/ Imperial Research Programme. When was that, way back in 1998?

AF: No, it was a long way after that. I set up the Beckley Foundation in 1998 in order to do scientific research and discover the mechanisms that underlie changes in consciousness. Then in 2005 I initiated a collaboration with professor David Nutt at Bristol, and that in time became the Beckley/Imperial Research Programme—in 2009. Things move very slowly. Now, finally, a shift is happening.

RLM: Given that Albert Hofmann discovered LSD in 1938, I believe.

AF: That was the first time, but then no one recognized that it had any interesting effects. Do you know the story? It's rather amazing. The first LSD was discarded, as it was tested on animals, and no obvious benefits were noted. Then, five years later, he resynthesized it, as a result of a "peculiar presentiment," namely that it might have other unknown effective qualities . . . something he'd never done for another compound. Then, somehow, he accidentally ingested some of the compound. That was in 1943. That is when the first LSD experience happened. He recognized the experience from mystical experiences in his youth.

RLM: That's what is referred to as the Bicycle Trip, isn't it?

AF: I think actually that was a few days later, when he took what he thought was the smallest dose you can take, 250 micrograms, which in fact turned out to be a very big trip, and it gave him quite an uncomfortable ride.

RLM: That was '43.

AF: Yes.

RLM: Then fast forward to 1966, when LSD was made illegal in the United States.

AF: Actually, I think federal law banned it in 1968, following the summer of love in '67.

RLM: Were you already doing research prior to 1966, or did your work start after that?

AF: In England it became illegal a bit later. I'd been studying mysticism and comparative religions, which had been my passion. Then I first took LSD in 1965, and in 1966 I met a Dutch scientist who had a new hypothesis of the mechanisms underlying changes in consciousness. It was then that I became fascinated with the scientific explanation of consciousness and how we could better understand it. It became my passion to do scientific research with it to explore these issues.

RLM: If you recall, tell us a little bit about your experience in 1965. The reason I'm asking for that is I want to put into context what we're going to be leading up to. Our listeners will hear some of the history, but what we're going to be leading up to is your recent groundbreaking research showing digital images of the inside of a brain on LSD and the placebo group that was not on LSD. Right now, we're going to hear about Amanda Feilding's first experience with this material, LSD, back in 1965 when it was still very legal in 1965 in England. Tell us about that experience, please.

AF: It was obviously an amazing experience, as people who've taken psychoactive substances know. It changes your visual experience and the way you hear music, and it provides a sense of wonder and unity. I, at that point, didn't think it was a way of life. It was more of a wonderful trip to the fun fair. Then the following year I met this scientist named Bart Huges, who had a hypothesis about how it changes the cerebral circulation, increasing the volume of blood in the brain capillaries. He explained that with this knowledge you could control your experience on LSD and use it as a tool with which to increase your cognitive functioning, creativity, and productivity, apart from of course having transformational experiences, insights, and a sense of union and connectivity with the universe.

RLM: He was already hypothesizing back in the '60s about blood flow and oxygen being regulated by this medicine.

AF: Exactly.

RLM: Lysergic acid diethylamide.

AF: Yes.

LSD and Changes in Consciousness

Whole Brain Communication

AF: His other major hypothesis, which I found of even greater interest, described the ego as a mechanism of constriction that is superimposed upon the rest of the brain and is developed by conditioning from infancy onward, becoming the controller of the gates of consciousness. It decides what gets through to consciousness and what is repressed. Amazingly, that is what our recent brain-imaging studies with psilocybin and LSD have shown. In modern neuroscientific terms it's called the "default mode network," a top-down controlling network that, interestingly, has its blood supply reduced by psychedelics so that its repressing function is reduced, the brain becomes more anarchical, and the whole brain begins to communicate.

Increased Blood Supply for Expanded Consciousness

RLM: When this gentleman that you met way back then was talking about controlling, was he talking about our being able to voluntarily take control of the blood flow to different areas of the brain in order to get through this gatekeeper that we're referring to as the ego?

AF: He described how the underlying action of a psychedelic substance is to constrict the veins, thereby increasing the volume of blood in the brain capillaries. Since the cranial cavity is a finite size it can only accept a larger volume of blood in the capillaries if an equal amount of cerebrospinal fluid—the other fluid volume in the brain—is squeezed out. By having more blood in the capillaries, there is more exchange of glucose and oxygen between the blood supply and brain cells. Likewise more waste products can be washed away. By changing the ratio between blood and cerebrospinal fluid in favor of blood, billions more brain cells are provided with sufficient energy to function simultaneously, and hence the expansion of consciousness one experiences on a psychedelic.

Bypassing the Ego Reflex Mechanism

AF: That is the basic hypothesis. The second hypothesis is about the "ego" being a reflex mechanism that is controlled through conditioning, and which then directs the blood where it is most needed. This ego mechanism controls the distribution of blood in the brain, and what becomes conscious and what does not. In a normal everyday situation, because of man's upright position and the skull closing at the end of growth, there is less blood in the brain than is optimal. When the blood supply to the brain is increased through a psychedelic substance, then connectivity throughout the brain is also increased. Remarkably, that is what we are seeing in our recent brain-imaging studies of the human brain on LSD.

RLM: Remarkably, what you're finding now, some fifty years later, is what this gentleman was hypothesizing to you as a young woman in your twenties, back in the 1960s.

AF: Yes. It is funny how long it has taken to get to this point. Of course, we could have been there twenty years ago if it wasn't for the fact that politics obstruct science.

RLM: You listened to this scientist. You've had one experience in 1965 with this material.

AF: I had many more than one experience.

RLM: After the first one?

AF: Yes.

RLM: You've had more than one experience. You're listening to this scientist. He's giving you some hypotheses about how this medicine that you've now taken more than once works. How does that affect you? How does that affect the course of your life after that?

AF: It actually very much changed the course of my life. I had had a passionate interest, as I said, in mystics and the mysticism that underlies spiritual and religious practices. I studied under the leading professor of the time, Professor R. C. Zaehner of All Souls College in Oxford. I was fascinated with and wanted to understand the unifying experience that all religions hold at their center. Then when I experienced LSD, I realized, "Wow this is it. Aha! This is the experience that the mystics talk about." For me, the description of the changes in blood supply—and how one could control those experiences by maintaining a normal glucose level in the blood—was very revealing.

The whole idea of the ego as this conditioned reflex mechanism that creates a veil between our perception of reality and actual reality through the veil of words made a lot of sense. I thought, this is so fascinating I will dedicate my life to researching more about it. I consider the study of consciousness to be the holy grail of scientific research. What is more important than a better understanding of our own consciousness? To be able to modulate the levels at which one is conscious is surely a very valuable new skill. This skill, of course, is not new, because obviously people have been doing it since the beginning of human civilization.

RLM: The search for consciousness and to understand consciousness indeed has been going on since the beginning.

AF: Yes.

Psychedelics Shake Up Rigid Patterns

RLM: Again, here you are. You're a young woman in your twenties. It's the 1960s. You're in England. You see this as a life changer.

AF: Yes.

RLM: What do you do?

AF: I more or less devoted the next fifty years to this topic. For the first forty years it was totally taboo! Now it is less of a taboo, I hope partly due to my labors. I think at last, hopefully, society is beginning to recognize that these compounds are extremely valuable as tools to alter consciousness and to be able to study consciousness and that they can open up amazing new avenues of treatment for many of our most debilitating illnesses such as depression, anxiety, addiction, post-traumatic stress disorder [PTSD], and OCD, among others.

All of these conditions are based on rigid thought patterns and behavioral patterns. What our studies show is that under the influence of a psychedelic, these rigid patterns are shaken. They lose their grip. By losing their grip, there's an afterglow once the psychedelic wears off.

United States' Political Influence

RLM: Amanda, I want to ask you a very personal question. I know that you are connected to the highest levels of English government. It's well known that you're part of the nobility; you're a countess yourself. My question is why do you think the English government has made this medicine illegal, and why do you think the English government has made basic scientific research at the very highest levels so difficult to do? What is your thinking? Why is that going on, please?

AF: To please America, to put it in the shortest possible way. It's a disgrace, because actually David Cameron, before becoming prime minister, was in favor of reform, quite clearly, and spoke very well on it, saying more or less the same things that I've been saying. When he became prime minister, all of that was forgotten, and sadly his home secretary, Theresa May, only a month ago brought about a new act that prohibited and criminalized *all* psychoactive substances, even those to be made in the future.

Sadly, she's just become our new prime minister. I would like to think that she will mend her ways and have a more thoughtful attitude. Maybe she will. Let's hope so.

RLM: Do you think she's coming from a place of concern about the United States government's attitude if she thinks differently, or do you think it's personal with her? What is your thinking about where she is coming from?

AF: I think she comes from probably a rather conventional, fearful, Middle England background on these issues. She's probably genuinely fearful of psychoactive substances. But she should know from studying the literature and from what's happening in other countries that if you want to protect the health of your children, and the children of the country, it's much better to legally regulate these substances, take them out of the hands of criminals, and bring them into the hands of educated, government-sponsored systems where they're regulated. One does one's very best to minimize harm and protect children from use before a suitable age and to educate and provide treatment for those who get in the habit of misusing them.

I became involved in this fight back in '98, and then there was no scientific evidence about the negative effects of illegal drugs. I set about trying to create an evidence-base, and now eighteen years later there is very firm evidence that shows that strong prohibition actually results in greater harm than from the drugs themselves. Countries like Portugal, which have decriminalized all drugs, have a much lower rate of use and, more importantly, of harmful use. It's going against the scientific evidence-base to be prohibitionist. America is changing within states, but the cruel thing is that the United Nations is completely controlled by the United States, and the UN controls all the countries in the world. All around the world, countries are having to keep psychoactive substances criminalized, whereas the United States of America can break their own conventions, and now their fastest growing industry is cannabis!

RLM: What is the prevalent thinking within the English government about why the United States government has continued to suppress scientific research in this particular area? How do the English see us about this?

AF: Actually, in the constitution of the UN, scientific and medical research is permitted. Sadly, the reality is that it's made impossible. Firstly, it's made so restrictive and so expensive that no one can undertake the research. Secondly, there's no funding. No one wants to fund the research, because they think it might be bad for their reputation. Thirdly, no scientist wants to get near it, because again it could damage their careers and future funding potential. For fifty years, there's been virtually no research on this incredibly valuable area of potential treatment. Now, luckily, because of the endeavors of a few small organizations like my own—the Beckley Foundation, Heffter, MAPS, and a few institutions like Johns Hopkins—it's slowly becoming apparent that these substances can actually bring about remarkable results.

I think that this reality is slowly beginning to permeate public consciousness. I've always thought that it's only through the very best scientific research that we have any hope of reintegrating these compounds into the fabric of society.

RLM: I totally agree with you that it's only the best scientific research that is going to educate us and show us what is possible. The question we come back to over and over again is a question that you've dedicated your life to promoting: How do we open the doors to allowing the research? That's why I'm coming back to the question of how English leaders view the United States and its sanctioning countries around the world who try to do this research.

I went to Israel some years ago with Rick Doblin, PhD, the founder of MAPS, and a group of scientists including Michael Mithoefer, PhD, who did the groundbreaking MDMA study that MAPS sponsored. While we were in Israel I was told by the head of their Supreme Court, "We would love to do this MDMA research with our post-traumatic stress disorder people, but we can't, because the United States government will sanction us if we do."

AF: Absolutely.

RLM: You're validating that in England it's the same feeling?

AF: Yes.

RLM: You're educating us that it goes beyond England, and that the United States government has used its power in the United Nations to suppress research worldwide. The question in 2016 again is, what do the English think the Americans are up to in suppressing research around the world? Do they think we're just crazy? Do they think there's a reason behind it? What do they think? Are we just a country gone nuts that we suppress science? What do you all think about us?

AF: What I think about it is one thing, but the government doesn't think about it at all.

RLM: They don't even think about it?

AF: They don't think about it. It's not a topic that interests them. It doesn't get votes in Middle England. Actually the interesting thing is the Americans—the U.S. government—have patented most of the cannabinoids while simultaneously criminalizing them. Way back in the '70s, they were patenting them.

RLM: Yes.

AF: It's a very dirty business, actually. The whole war on drugs has caused untold suffering in countries around the world under the pretense that it's to protect young people from drugs. Actually, the U.S. government had a whole load of different reasons for getting the war on drugs into other countries, such as controlling socio-political situations. It's done more damage I think than any other civil intervention.

RLM: Political influence, of course.

AF: Yeah.

RLM: In this country we've got our prisons and jails disproportionately full of young black men who have been put away for relatively minor marijuana offenses.

AF: Absolutely. I think you are seven times more likely to go to prison if you're black than if you're white, and no more blacks use these substances than whites. It's appalling. It's the same in England. It's a new form of discrimination.

RLM: Yeah, we learned that in *Chasing the Scream.** I know you know the author, Johann Hari.

AF: Absolutely.

RLM: We have this painful situation. Our prisons and jails are full here. We have more people in jail I think than . . .

AF: Than any other country in the world.

RLM: Everybody knows that about us.

AF: Yes. Isn't it the biggest growing industry in California?

RLM: The industry of institutionalization of people who have been convicted for minor offenses.

AF: Yes.

RLM: It's a horror story.

AF: Yes.

Birthing Brain Cells with Ayahuasca

RLM: Within that horror story we're going to come back to your breakthrough research that you were able to do after lifelong pushing, and we want to hear about it. Please tell us something about a topic that's exotic to a lot of listeners: your research with ayahuasca.

AF: Yes, that's very recent. We collaborated with a researcher in Barcelona called Jordi Riba, and he's probably the leading researcher on ayahuasca in the world. Together, we have carried out a series of studies with ayahuasca, and this particular one you are referring to was looking at whether compounds in ayahuasca produce the birth of new brain cells.

---

*Johann Hari, *Chasing the Scream: The First and Last Days of the War on Drugs* (New York: Bloomsbury USA, 2015).

RLM: The actual birth of new brain cells.

AF: Yes, it was done in a petri dish, with cells from the hippocampus of mice. It's quite amazing how we saw a flood of new neurons.

RLM: I'm looking at one of your slides as you speak. I'm actually looking at a slide of young neurons, they're stained green, and then mature neurons, they're stained red. It's a beautiful piece of work here, by the way. Thank you so much for it.

AF: Isn't it exciting? It's literally a very first phase, but as we all know many illnesses like dementia and Alzheimer's result from the death of brain cells. We know now that new neurons can be made in the adult brain, which ten years ago scientists didn't think could happen. This is a flood of new neurons. If this can be replicated in vivo, it could be a great step forward in the research of novel treatments for neurodegenerative diseases. I would be surprised if we didn't find that other psychoactive substances also stimulate the birth of new neurons. That's something I very much want to investigate next, to see if LSD might have the same effect.

LSD's Burst of Connectivity

RLM: I want to discuss the study that was recently written up in the *New York Times* with photographs of your brain imaging. Please tell us about your digital-imaging research with LSD.

AF: Yes. That's very exciting. My old passion from the '60s was investigating the changes in cerebral circulation underlying the changes in neural functioning brought about by LSD. The study we published in April and presented at the Royal Society in London shows how the visual parts of the brain act in normal circumstances, that is, on the placebo. Then, when the infusion of LSD takes place, one sees suddenly the whole brain is much more connected. Different parts of the brain are speaking to each other simultaneously. The whole brain is lit up with connectivity—the blood supply is increased.

There is a burst of connectivity, which goes a long way in explaining why, when on LSD, one has the feeling that one's seeing is much, much deeper. You see beauty with incredible depth, and it's the same with music. Everyone has always said how amazingly deep, vibrant, and wonderful musical and visual stimulations are when using LSD. That's because the parts of the brain that are dealing with emotion and memory are all talking with the visual areas. They are informing the visual area. Indeed, we can now see the mechanisms of hallucinations, in that there is as much stimulation of the visual area of the brain with eyes closed as with eyes open.

RLM: I'm looking at a slide from your research, and it's so dramatic. I'm looking at the slide of the brains from the subjects who had taken the LSD, and it's bright. The whole brain is bright and lit up.

AF: Absolutely.

RLM: Remember folks, these slides were made by functional magnetic resonance imaging [fMRI]. We actually are looking at the inside of the brain, and I'm looking at photographs of these slides. The placebo subjects, who received no LSD, have little patches of lit up areas, but most of the brain is dark.

AF: Yes, absolutely.

RLM: It's as if this is validating the stuff that we've been hearing all our lives on the street, which is that you only use 5 percent of your brain, or you only use 10 percent of it. It turns out, according to your research, that's accurate.

AF: Yes, we certainly don't use our brains optimally. That's what's so incredibly exciting. That's really why I set up the Beckley Foundation, because with brain imaging you can actually see what's happening in the brain at the same time as the person is having an experience, and it can tell you what is underlying the experience. That is, you can correlate the experience with changes in brain activity. Really, the combination of brain imaging and psychedelic substances, which alter consciousness in such a reliable and profound way, is an incredible microscope to the workings of the mind. The impact of brain imaging and psychedelics for the study of consciousness is comparable to the impact of the telescope to astronomy and the microscope to biology.

RLM: Again, it's bringing us back to what your friend theorized some fifty years ago, that the LSD is evidently opening up the vessels so that the brain areas that are ordinarily not used are being infused with more oxygen, which allows those areas to be utilized.

AF: And glucose.

RLM: Oxygen and glucose.

AF: Consciousness is the result of the oxidation of glucose, the energy that produces the neuronal activity. Just last week I embarked on a new study, which is very exciting. It's been a well-known fact for quite a few years now that LSD, and indeed all psychedelics, works through the serotonin 2A receptor. Nobody knows what happens beyond that. With a new form of optogenetics investigation, one can see right into the pyramidal cells, which are found in layer five of the cortex, and see how they react to LSD and how changes in the blood supply are related to the stimulation of neurons. We can work out which comes first—whether changes in blood supply stimulate neurons, or whether the stimulation of neurons creates changes in blood supply. Which is the egg and which is the chicken?

RLM: We have a combination of possibilities here. It is so exciting talking to you. You bring us the possibility of actually taking a medicine that will create new neurons, bringing more activity into play. At the same time, another medicine may stimulate cerebral circulation and neuronal activity and allow us to actually access other areas of our brain that we haven't had access to on a day-to-day basis as we go through life. As you've explained to us, we grow what you call filters as we're living and the filters constrict us.

AF: Yes, the building up of the constricting, filtering mechanism is an incredible process that happens in humans particularly, from infancy onward, as we slowly learn the art of control and repression. Obviously, it's a vital element that enables us to do all the incredible things we do. At the same time it can become a very dangerous implementation that can stop us from having a real grasp of reality, because we're looking through a veil of words and superimposed meaning, which may have little relationship with reality.

RLM: Our greatest asset becomes our greatest liability, as is so often the case.

AF: Absolutely, and as we get older this kind of set pattern of behavior—the one-track thinking, the myopic vision—becomes more and more established. In fact when it gets really rigid, this rigidity underlies conditions like depression, and addiction, and obsessive-compulsive disorders, all of those conditions that are based on hyper, fixed patterns of thought and behavior. That's what a psychedelic experience seems to shake in a way that actually leaves an afterglow. Actually this is all kind of new, these findings with the recent research. It's very exciting to see. It allows us to see how these compounds work in the brain and their value.

In the last fifty years I've met many, many people who've said, "My goodness. I would have never done this without the insights I had through my LSD experience," whether it was starting a school in India for untouchable children or discovering DNA [like Kary Mullis]. It wasn't obvious why or what the mechanisms underlying these experiences were. That's what we are beginning to unravel now.

I think our foot is only just in the door, but it's a lovely place to be, *in the door*. It's much better than being outside the door, which is where we have been, in terms of understanding the mechanisms underlying consciousness.

RLM: Definitely. Twice during our interview you've mentioned this afterglow. You used the word *afterglow* after taking the medicine. Elaborate a little bit for us on this afterglow that you're talking about.

AF: That's like what is shown in the depression study: that three months later 42 percent of the study patients are still experiencing a remission in chronic depression, and they're still reporting feeling much more optimistic and having more of a sense of openness. In the research I've done with Jordi Riba with ayahuasca, people report the same thing—much more openness. Also, there are measures of mindfulness that people can gain through mindful meditation. People who are regular ayahuasca users score a high level of mindfulness on these tests.

There's a very fascinating observation we made in our first psilocybin study, which was about this network in the brain called the "default mode network," which has only recently been identified. In a way it's like the conductor in an orchestra. It's part of the ego mechanism described by Freud, which controls what enters consciousness and what doesn't. It's a circuit of high-level hub centers that control the sensory perceptions coming in, determining whether they get through to consciousness or whether they're repressed and kept beneath the threshold of consciousness. It's like the controller of the veils, basically.

On a psychedelic—in this case it was psilocybin—we noticed that there was a reduction in blood flow to the default mode network. What we noticed was that the integrity within the network disappeared. Usually within a network there's a lot of communication between the different key hubs. In the default mode network there are two very important hubs: one is the medial prefrontal cortex and the other is the posterior cingulate cortex.

In depressed patients it had been observed that there is chronic over-activity between these two centers. There is a repetitive conversation saying, "I'm so depressed, I'm so depressed," or "I want another drink, I want another drink." When the psychedelic reduces the blood supply to this network, the activity drops. The controlling grip of the default mode network diminishes. Suddenly, all the different networks in the brain begin to communicate with each other. These networks, which were normally anticorrelated, that is, didn't talk to each other, suddenly begin talking. That's what we can see in the LSD study. We have all these different parts in the brain lit up, communicating with each other.

RLM: You are conducting the pioneering work on understanding the mechanism that's going on in the brain in relation to the psychedelic medicines.

AF: Exactly. That's the action beneath the mystical experience—when the person experiences themselves as being part of the whole, part of the universe, part of however they want to verbalize it.

Not Addictive Medicines

RLM: We've got a little time left. I want to ask a couple of quick questions, Amanda. One is, I've had a specialty of addiction treatment going back for many decades, and I've treated people for heroin and cocaine addiction. I don't get people coming in addicted to LSD or to psilocybin or ayahuasca. Why is that?

AF: Because they simply aren't addictive. You cannot make an animal addicted to a psychedelic. They are nontoxic and nonaddictive.

RLM: They're not only nontoxic, they're also nonaddictive.

AF: Yeah.

Voluntary Healing?

RLM: Next question. When we cut ourselves and healing takes place—like on the back of my arm, if I cut myself it would heal—it's involuntary. It just happens. Do you think that with these medicines there will be a day when we'll be able to take voluntary control of our healing? Will we be able to focus the mind in such a way that rather than all healing being involuntary, we'll be able to go inside, find damaged tissue on an organ, and actually use the mind to aid in the repair voluntarily? Can you see that happening?

AF: Possibly. That's a power that high-level yogis have. I think it's a very high-level skill. But if it is possible, psychedelics could help to achieve it, with much trained concentration.

RLM: Do you think the medicines that you're researching can assist us in learning how to take voluntary control of our mind toward healing and repair?

AF: I do, and I also think they can assist in taking the blood supply to repressed areas. I think the core of a trauma is a repressed area, which is cut off from freely moving blood circulation. The pain is locked into this "do not enter" area. By removing the repression in this area—which is brought about by the default mode network protecting the person against the pain—by washing it out, you can wash out the pain, and then the repressed area can heal itself. I think these substances are amazing tools of healing, but also of self-realization and transformation. They are also tools for creativity, because they enable different parts of the brain to work simultaneously, allowing new combinations of ideas to come together.

In many ways they're a win-win gift. They're a gift of the gods that modern man has foolishly criminalized. It's time that we left this dark age, and we integrate psychedelics with the knowledge of science, medicine, and spirituality. I think finally the tide has begun to turn, and hopefully, we're slowly climbing that particular mountain.

RLM: Thank you, Amanda Feilding. Thank you for your lifework and for bringing us out of this darkness of lack of research. Thank you for putting so much of your time, energy, and lifework into bringing research out to the public so that these medicines will eventually become available, and thank you so much for appearing on our program today. It's been a pleasure having you.

AF: Thank you very, very much. Let's hope governments can change and allow us to set up clinics where people can get this therapy.

RLM: Hear, hear!

•••

Four Thousand Journeys

Our next expert in the field of LSD research is Stanislav Grof, MD, PhD, a Czech psychiatrist, one of the founders of the field of transpersonal psychology, and a researcher into the use of nonordinary states of consciousness for purposes of exploring, healing, and obtaining growth and insights into the human psyche. Dr. Grof had the good fortune to have been around while LSD was still legal. This allowed him to do direct psychotherapy with LSD. We have the good fortune that he recorded much of his work, publishing many books on the topic (see his biography). While reading the interview, keep in mind that Stan has guided people in over four thousand LSD journeys, probably more than any other person on the planet.

Observations from 4,000 LSD Sessions
Stanislav Grof, MD, PhD
July 21, 2015

STANISLAV GROF, MD, PHD, is author of *Realms of the Human Unconscious, LSD Psychotherapy, Beyond Death, The Adventure of Self Discovery, Beyond the Brain, Psychology of the Future, The Cosmic Game, Healing Our Deepest Wounds,* and *Modern Consciousness Research and the Understanding of Art.*

A Package from Albert Hofmann to Stanislav Graf

Abandoning Freudian Therapy for Cartooning

RLM: You started out as a psychiatrist doing Freudian work. You were initially deeply interested in psychoanalysis, but then something happened that brought you into the field of research with LSD.

Stanislav Grof, MD, PhD (SG): I was born in Prague, Czechoslovakia, and originally wanted to go into animated movies. Just before I made the final commitment, I read *Freud's Introductory Lectures on Psychoanalysis* and I got very excited. That week I decided not to work in animated movies but to study medicine and to become a psychiatrist. As I was getting deeper into psychoanalysis I became disappointed—at first not with the theory but with the practice of psychoanalysis: how long it takes, how much money it costs, and how much energy it consumes. And the results were not exactly breathtaking. I started nostalgically returning in my mind to animated movies, feeling that it would have been a better career.

Then the psychiatric department I was working in received a large supply of LSD-25 from the pharmaceutical company Sandoz in Basel, Switzerland. It came with a letter describing the serendipitous discovery of its psychedelic effect by Albert Hofmann, a chemist who intoxicated himself accidentally when he was synthesizing it. It was supposed to be one of the substances used in gynecology and for relief of migraine headaches, which were the main indications of the ergot alkaloids, though Hofmann's discovery was a very unexpected fringe benefit from this research. It was not considered a particularly interesting substance, so the research was discontinued. Those of us who knew Albert Hofmann frequently heard the story that he somehow could not get this substance off his mind for irrational reasons. He felt the pharmacologists must have overlooked something. So in 1943 he decided to synthesize another sample and this is when the intoxication occasion happened.

RLM: Yes, the famous bicycle ride.

An Unconventional Experimental Tool

RLM: So Sandoz sent LSD around the world, and you were one of the people to whom it was sent. You received the package, and what happened?

SG: The letter accompanying the package suggested on the basis of the pilot studies conducted in Zurich that LSD could be used for inducing experimental psychosis. We would have a model that we could study. There was another suggestion that this could be a kind of unconventional educational tool—that psychiatrists, psychologists, nurses, and students would have the chance to spend a few hours in a world that seemed to be like the world of some of their patients. This would help them to understand their patients better, to be able to communicate with them more effectively and hopefully be more successful in treating them. That was something that was sorely needed at the time; psychiatric therapy was truly medieval—electroshock, insulin comas, cardiazol shocks, dunking in cold water, straitjackets, and so forth.

RLM: So the therapists would have an experiential understanding of the psychoses of their patients by going into that realm for a limited number of hours?

SG: Yes, that was the idea. At that point I was quite disappointed with psychoanalysis, and this seemed like a new possibility. I became an early volunteer in Prague, and I had an experience that within a day transformed me professionally and personally.

Transformation from Materialist to Mystic

RLM: I heard you talk about that transformation at the Bently Reserve presentation. How can you start out as Stan Grof, take a substance, and at the end of the experience be a different Stan Grof?

SG: I was brought up in a family where there was no religious affiliation. My parents did not commit me or my brother to any religion. I had a very materialistic worldview and went from this family upbringing straight to medical school, which certainly does not cultivate mystical awareness. Czechoslovakia was at that time controlled by the Soviet Union, and we had a very strong materialistic education. Yet within those few hours in this experience I basically became somebody with a spiritual, mystical worldview and a completely transformed perspective on life. Also, my interest shifted from psychoanalysis to nonordinary states of consciousness. Research into these states has now been for over half a century my profession, my vocation, and I would say *passion*. I have done very little in this half century that has not been related to these special states of consciousness.

RLM: Talk to us more about this transition. What does it mean to be a materialist, and what does it mean to you to be more spiritual or mystical?

SG: I was trained to believe that this was a material universe, which in a sense created itself without any guiding intelligence. There was no place for spirituality. If we believe that this is a universe of matter and that life, intelligence, and consciousness are latecomers after billions of years of the development of matter, then they are just side products or "epiphenomena" of material processes. This worldview rejected spirit; to be spiritual meant to be ignorant and superstitious, not having studied what material science discovered and says about the universe.

This was a completely different perspective than one saying the universe is permeated by superior intelligence and that consciousness is a fundamental aspect of the universe—not the side product of the human brain. It was a very radical transformation.

RLM: Are you putting forth that there is a consciousness floating through the universe? Perhaps some Möbius strip of consciousness that is always around us? How do you conceptualize this spiritual consciousness?

SG: Consciousness for us is like water for fish. It is a fundamental aspect of our existence. If I had to name an existing conceptual framework for what I have experienced, I would go to the great spiritual philosophies of the East: Hinduism, Buddhism, and Taoism. These cultures were involved in systematic exploration of consciousness, with the same kind of focus and enthusiasm that we have for the material world. They were not particularly interested in developing technologies and industry. Their focus was on exploration of consciousness. Their understanding of the human psyche and consciousness was way beyond what we have now in the materialistic science in the West.

A New Worldview
Curbing Our Rationality and Connecting with Nature

RLM: I'm beginning to understand what you mean by being transformed in a day. Starting out with a materialistic framework has political implications for how we live our lives in terms of the importance of acquiring material things and living in a culture that values material things as the goal. It is light years away from a conceptual framework in which spirituality and consciousness are paramount. Therefore, the value system that would come out of a spiritual world-view would be much more aligned with feelings and people—in terms of their nature and in terms of connecting with nature rather than connecting with things. Is that correct?

SG: Yes. We have now the most advanced worldview in Western science—the new or emerging paradigm—and we see that it is rapidly converging with this spiritual worldview of ancient systems, particularly the great spiritual philosophies and religions of the Far East. There are repeated reports now from quantum relativistic physics that come to the same conclusion—that consciousness is somehow fundamentally involved in the creation of the experience of the material world itself.

RLM: Yes.

SG: The new science is converging with mysticism. What we were experiencing and finding in our psychedelic research was fundamentally incompatible with the Cartesian-Newtonian worldview—basically the seventeenth-century philosophy—but perfectly reconcilable with the emerging paradigm.

Observations from 4,000 LSD Sessions
Peeling the Unconscious

RLM: Some time after you had this transformation, you moved to the United States.

SG: Yes. I had my first psychedelic session in 1956, and I moved to the United States in 1967. I had worked in psychedelic research in Prague for eleven years before leaving the country.

RLM: Were you able to do LSD research during those eleven years?

SG: Yes. We were doing something that we called psycholytic therapy, which was a large number of medium dosages of LSD—something that one of my patients called "onion peeling of the unconscious." We were able to remove layer after layer and map the unconscious, moving from the Freudian individual, or personal unconscious, through what I call "the perinatal unconscious," related to the memory of birth, to what Jung called the collective unconscious—both its historical and mythological, or archetypal, aspects.

RLM: During that period, Stan, from 1956 to 1967—eleven years—approximately how many people were treated with this dosage of LSD?

SG: If I add up the sessions in Prague and later in the United States, I have been personally involved in about four thousand psychedelic sessions.

RLM: What is a medium dose?

SG: Maybe about 150 to 200 micrograms. Once we go to 250 and up to 500 micrograms, we would call them high-dose sessions.

Neither Panacea nor Devil's Drug

RLM: The American public has been, one might say, traumatized by the very word LSD as a result of the terrible negative publicity that came out of the 1960s. But here we have someone who has done actual scientific research—four thousand cases—to tell us whether this is a dangerous medicine. Are the side effects such that your patients were jumping out of windows? Did they have to be institutionalized?

SG: Well, it is a very powerful tool. The perspectives ranged from calling it a panacea to the devil's drug. What is overlooked is that this is a tool. Humphry Osmond [the English psychiatrist and researcher who coined the term psychedelic] compared it to a knife. Is a knife a terribly dangerous tool or is it a useful instrument? Imagine a discussion where the chief of the New York Police Department would describe the murders committed in the back streets of New York City, and the Surgeon General would say, "Well, if you have the right kind of education you can do amazing medical interventions with the knife." And we would have in the same discussion a housewife talk, who would think about a knife primarily as a tool to cut salami and vegetables, and an artist whose emphasis would be using it for carving wood. It would be absolutely clear that we are not talking about the knife—we are talking about the various *human* uses of the knife for different purposes and different intentions.

Psychedelics were used for many different reasons—from therapy of difficult psychiatric patients and alleviation of fear of death and physical pain in terminal cancer patients, through facilitation of mystical experiences or artistic inspiration, to means of compromising of foreign diplomats and chemical warfare. What would happen if you put it into people's water supply? If you would use it in aerosols in the field? If you would smuggle it somehow into the drinks of diplomats and politicians and military leaders and so on? Those are all human uses with very different motivations. Psychedelics are powerful openers of the mind, so they can be used for all those different purposes. So it is a question of set and setting—who is giving psychedelics to whom, in what physical environment, with what kind of intention, and for what kind of purpose.

In industrial civilization we have so far abused everything. We have abused biology for biological warfare, chemistry for chemical warfare, atomic energy for nuclear warfare, laser and rockets for destructive purposes, and so on. Why would psychedelics be different? We are incredibly developed in terms of the neocortex and intellectual capacity, but we stayed stuck in the Stone Age with our emotion. As a result, we are using nuclear weapons and other means of mass destruction with the same kind of mentality with which the Neanderthals were using stones and sticks.

Understanding Our
Ecological Interconnectedness

RLM: Well, there is a reason that LSD has such a psychological effect on the public: the fact that the medicine itself can change consciousness; for example, your experience of starting out as one Stan Grof, with a materialistic framework for how the world works, and then achieving a new Stan Grof, with a different worldview: expanded from materialism to spiritualism plus mysticism. That is a radical transformation. This medicine could be seen, and I think it is seen by many, as revolutionary, because it has the potential to change consciousness on a grand scale; is that not accurate?

SG: It has tremendous potential for individual therapy, but it is also associated with a radical transformation of worldview and bringing in the spiritual perspective. If it could be applied on a large enough scale, it could significantly increase our chances for survival on the planet. If we continue our ignorant strategy—bringing a linear focus into a biological system that is basically circular—we do not have great chances for survival. Plundering of nonrenewable resources and turning them into pollution is the last thing we need as biological entities. We need clean water, clean air, and clean soil in which we grow our food. Nothing is more important—no economic, political, ideological, military, or religious concerns. Nothing should be more important than protecting life and creating optimal conditions for survival on the planet. We are violating this and are polluting the very environment that we depend on.

This can change through these transformative experiences, where people can work through the traumas that they experienced in childhood, in infancy, during birth and prenatal existence. We need to be open to the mystical, spiritual perspective—recognizing our fundamental connection with other people and the way we are embedded in nature. We cannot do anything to harm nature that will not ricochet and hurt us.

Caution Required

RLM: We have millions of people in the United States, and I do not know how many around the world, who are experimenting on their own with LSD. We do not have alarming reports from emergency rooms around the United States about mass occurrences of psychotic breakdowns. We do not have reports from police departments around the United States of incidents being created by LSD. These people are taking it on their own as you well know—as we all well know. Some of them have guides, some of them do not have guides. They are taking this substance that has huge potential for transformation. Why are we not hearing more, over these decades, about emergency room incidents, and police, and people killing people?

SG: There was a big study conducted by Sidney Cohen, one of the early pioneers.

RLM: I remember him—yes.

SG: A psychoanalyst in Los Angeles. He wrote a review of the side effects and complications of LSD and mescaline sessions, drawn from twenty-five thousand administrations.* The side effects and negative aftereffects were minimal as long as it was done responsibly. In the early years, we did not know very much about the effects of these psychedelics, but it was understood that if somebody had this powerful experience, there had to be somebody around in the usual state of consciousness to "hold the kite string." You had to keep people overnight and talk with them in the morning before you sent them home. Under those circumstances the incidence of complications was minimal. It was ridiculous compared with what we had with electroshocks or insulin comas, where 1 percent mortality was considered an acceptable therapeutic risk.

---

*Sidney Cohen, "Lysergic Acid Diethylamide: Side Effects and Complications," *Journal of Nervous and Mental Diseases* 130 (January 1960): 30–40.

RLM: Yes, or the lobotomy.

SG: Do you know that in 1948, Portuguese neurosurgeon Edgar Moniz was awarded the Nobel Prize for prefrontal lobotomy? Nobel Prize for lobotomy, where you insert a scalpel into the frontal lobe and cut it off. This was the original, massive lobotomy, not the refined transorbital lobotomy. I have seen in autopsies of these patients that an entire frontal lobe was changed into a large hemorrhagic cyst. All these were procedures with incredible risk compared to the responsible use of psychedelics. People were using psychedelics in places like Woodstock, where they were handing out all kinds of substances of unknown origin, quality, and dosages—handing it out with both hands. It is a miracle that there were not more complications under such circumstances, if we compare it with what can happen with alcohol.

Psychedelics are certainly powerful tools. It makes me very uncomfortable when I see that young people play with them in open public places where nobody is holding the space, knowing that they are doing something illegal and that police might show up any minute. This kind of use significantly increases the risks and diminishes potential benefits and gains. I hope that the recent renaissance of interest in psychedelic research will generate new unbiased information and eventually lead not only to mainstream therapeutic use but also eventually to the creation of a network of facilities where people who want to experiment with psychedelics will have the chance to do it with known doses of pharmaceutically pure substances and under expert guidance. This will take us far in the direction that Albert Hofmann wanted to see for LSD, his "wonder child" turned "problem child"—a New Atlantis in which psychedelics' potential for healing, enhancement of creativity, and spiritual opening will be integrated into future society and contribute to international peaceful coexistence.

•••

A Psychedelic Explorer

For my final interview on the topic of LSD, I am delighted to include Jim Fadiman, PhD, a colleague and a friend. I first met Jim in the late 1960s when we were both among a group of over two hundred psychologists that joined with Nick Cummings, PhD, who later became the president of the American Psychological Association, in starting the California School for Professional Psychology, the first independent, free-standing, PhD-granting, psychology graduate school in the United States. Jim is widely acknowledged for his extensive work in the field of psychedelic research, including a major contribution with his most recent book, *The Psychedelic Explorer's Guide.*

The Condensed Psychedelic Explorer's Guide
James Fadiman, PhD
October 18, 2011

JAMES FADIMAN, PHD, is a psychologist and author of *The Psychedelic Explorer's Guide: Safe, Therapeutic, and Sacred Journeys.* He is one of the foremost pioneers of the potential for psychedelic substances for self-discovery, psychotherapy, and creative problem solving and has been involved with psychedelic research since the 1960s. Fadiman is the president of the Association for Transpersonal Psychology and the director at the Institute of Noetic Sciences. He cofounded, along with Robert Frager, the Institute of Transpersonal Psychology, which later became Sofia University.

A Country of Hypocrites

RLM: How were you able to write a book, *The Psychedelic Explorer's Guide,* about exploring a medicine that is illegal to administer or use?

Jim Fadiman, PhD (JF): One way is to recognize that there is some basic research that we had started before the government stopped us, and there is some research that's coming back in. The other is to notice that since the government banned all possible use, including research, and so forth, 23 million Americans have taken LSD. And not only that, but that number goes up by four to six hundred thousand each year.

RLM: How does a researcher get those numbers?

JF: Personally, I think the numbers are a little low because they come from the U.S. government. Imagine the government gives you a little form and says, "Please check off all the illegal activities you have been involved in, in the last month, and in your lifetime." I suspect there is underreporting. And remember that's only the United States and that is only LSD. If we include MDMA, or ecstasy, the figure jumps by millions. If you simply add other consciousness-altering drugs, like marijuana, there are 140 million people in the United States who don't think prohibition personally applies to them. We are a country of lawbreakers, or as some people say, we're a country of plant users.

RLM: I suppose from another perspective we're a country of hypocrites.

JF: The people who make laws often do it based on spur-of-the-moment excitement. One of the reasons the research is coming back is the government actually is no longer desperately trying to prevent research, it's just allowing the research to proceed extremely carefully and safely.

Putting Real Dangers in Perspective

RLM: LSD. How dangerous is it? If you look at the sun while you're on LSD do you go blind? Does hair grow on the palm of your hands? Do you end up in the emergency room? We have now had forty to fifty years of people using it on their own, illegally. You're citing figures going into the tens of millions—you know how many people are being admitted to the emergency rooms each year around the country. You know how many people have died, so please share that information with us.

JF: I say to people that these are very powerful substances, and used incorrectly you can get in trouble. Used correctly, the chances of anything going wrong are extraordinarily low. One of the reasons I like LSD is that you use literally a hundred millionths of a gram—there are almost no physiological changes.

Things go wrong if you take it in the wrong setting, with the wrong friends, at the wrong time, with the wrong other substances. Or if you take too much—which is true of most other substances. Tobacco causes approximately 400,000 deaths a year. Alcohol causes approximately 125,000 deaths per year. Peanuts cause about 100 deaths. Psychedelics aren't even on the list. Although I am beginning to worry about peanuts. Have people gotten into serious trouble? Have some been hospitalized for years after taking psychedelics? The answer is yes, but probably as much from the bad situation and from the kind of well-meaning but ignorant health care they received immediately afterward.

Forbidden Fruit
and the Folly of Prohibition

JF: If you go to Burning Man, where there's a huge amount of drug use, they have a medical tent, and what they call Sanctuary, which is there to help people who are frightened, upset, and paranoid (also dehydrated), usually to simply recover without interrupting the flow, so the experience can complete itself. There are even ways to work with very difficult situations, which are especially common at major concerts or festivals, where people have not had the chance to get decent information for the last forty years. One of the reasons I wrote the book was to put out the basic safety information, to ensure that if people are going to use something illegally that they have the best information available—to get the safest and most beneficial experience possible. We must not forget that the reason people want to use these substances is because they feel there's some benefit.

RLM: Yes, so here we have a legal book about how to use an illegal substance, which is so attractive to people that they're using it by the tens of millions—right in the face of government and media focus that says: "This is so dangerous that we're making it illegal."

JF: The last time the government tried to prevent people from doing what they wanted was called Prohibition. Before Prohibition, there were eight hundred drinking establishments around Times Square. During Prohibition there were twenty-five hundred drinking establishments in that same area. We should have learned that prohibition is not the best way to prevent people from using whatever it is that the government doesn't like.

RLM: In fact, if anything, it makes it more interesting. It's like when we were told as children that we should keep away from a certain thing the adults might be using, and we were thinking, "Gee, if that's the thing to keep away from, I want to find out what it is."

JF: We must never give a bean to a small child and say, "Don't put it up your nose."

Six Variables for a Safe and Beneficial Psychedelic Session

RLM: I'm asking you a question I shouldn't ask, but I'm asking anyway—if you're allowed to do this, tell us, what is the proper way to take LSD?

JF: I'm going to give your listeners a premium. There are several chapters of the book up for free on EntheoGuide.net, which describe it in detail. They asked me to contribute those chapters so that people would have access to the six major variables that make a successful psychedelic session. Successful means healthy, safe, and meaningful. Those include:

First, the mental set.

Second, the physical setting, which should be safe and comfortable.

Third, the sitter—I *recommend, recommend, recommend* a guide who can assist you if you get into places that are frightening or difficult.

Fourth, the substance—there are many kinds of psychedelics and how much you take matters.

Fifth, the session itself—how the six to twelve hours run, what you do during that time.

Sixth, what kind of a life group you come back into—to people who support this kind of expanded awareness? Or to people who feel that you have just done something either evil or dangerous?

I want those basics available out there as widely as possible, because I'm a safety nut, and I'm also a guide nut. You don't learn to drive by throwing someone the car keys and saying, "Good luck!"

Set: Mental Attitude and Intention

RLM: What is set?

JF: Set is mental attitude or intention. Are you taking this because you would like to become closer to divinity, however you understand that? Or are you taking it because you are interested in working on your own personal issues? Or are you taking it just for self-discovery? Are you taking it just for recreation? Someone in New York recently asked me at a conference, "Is there anything wrong with using things just to have fun?" I had to admit there is a good argument for that. Other ways of using it are for scientific problem solving—for very hard-nosed, rational problems—and just for discovering what happens inside your own mind when you give it a nudge in a different direction.

RLM: What is an example of using LSD for problem solving?

JF: We did some research just as the government was shutting us down, and we'd had senior scientists taking what we call low doses of LSD. That would be 100 micrograms, a hundred millionth of a gram, and we basically gave them a safe, supportive setting. We gave them a couple of hours of free ranging inside their mind, and we then asked them at the peak of the experience to work on their own chosen problem—an important technical problem—and I mean very technical: theory of the photon, chip design, engineering problems, architecture problems, and so forth. Things that they had hitherto worked on and not been successful. That was our criteria, because we wanted them to care a lot about problem solving.

There's been a lot of stuff on every level about Steve Jobs, and my favorite headline is "Steve Jobs Had LSD. We Have the iPhone."* From what he reported, it was one of the most important experiences of his life. And to me that meant that he did it well—did it carefully. He was looking at the material world as well as his inner world.

RLM: We don't know whether he continued to use it, we just know that he did use it early on. There are so many people—as you well know, Jim, myself included at various times in my career—who were willing to talk about using it many years ago. If there are those who would prosecute me I would say, "That was thirty years ago."

---

*Maia Szalavitz, Time.com, October 6, 2011, http://healthland.time.com/2011/10/06 /jobs-had-lsd-we-have-the-iphone/ (accessed April 30, 2017).

JF: But I think we can say with Steve Jobs that we have zero indication that he used it later in his life. He did use it early in his life. It was part of what oriented him toward elegance, and beauty, and making things easy for people, but he did not use it and come up with the iPad.

RLM: But we also know, for example, that Carl Sagan's widow revealed he had used LSD but was afraid to tell the world. Even a man of his great magnitude was afraid to tell the world that he used it in some of those discoveries, which I think speaks volumes about the fear level that has been perpetrated in our country about this.

JF: Fear and social stigma. When I walk around carrying this book—as authors do—almost everyone I meet suddenly begins telling me about their psychedelic experiences after I talk to them for a while.

RLM: Jim Fadiman is referring to his book, *The Psychedelic Explorer's Guide: Safe, Therapeutic, and Sacred Journeys.* So we have some idea of what set means: your mental set, that is, what's going on in your mind—your intention.

Setting: Landscapes and Soundscapes

RLM: The next thing one wants to be aware of when experimenting with psychedelic medicine is setting. What is setting?

JF: Setting is literally the physical situation in which you find yourself. Albert Hofmann, who was still giving two-hour lectures to professional groups at 101 years old, was asked—as he said, "only ten thousand times"—how should you take LSD? His answer was, "Always take it in nature."

My answer is a little different. Take it in as safe and comfortable a setting as possible, which often is the living room, where you are able also to lie down to listen to music through headphones or earbuds; and to even put on an eye mask so that you can investigate the universe from the inside. Then perhaps later in the day it is good to be outside in nature to investigate the universe from the outside. Setting is the physical environment and the people who are in that environment—which we'll get to when we talk about sitter, because taking it around people you feel safe with turns out to be very important.

RLM: What about the place of ambient noise? Is that a factor that people should be cautious about? A machine noise, lawn mowers—the things that are going to intrude on consciousness?

JF: One of the wonderful things we have technologically are headphones, which block out ambient noise. Almost everyone, including indigenous people, find music or singing to be a very important part of the psychedelic experience. What we've found is, the reason people prefer music, and music without words, is that it allows them to stop thinking about daily trivia and to simply appreciate the enormous expansion of awareness that comes with almost any psychedelic. The most common comment we hear is, "I never knew music could be so beautiful and so intricate."

You know, when you hear a symphony orchestra, and you kind of hear a blur of sound with the melody rising and falling? If you're a professional musician you hear more, but on psychedelics, people report hearing each individual section, working with and against the others, and even report hearing individual players. So you're hearing with a much higher level of awareness. Headphones seemed to be the best way to handle the lawn mower, the ambulance, and the jackhammers.

RLM: So the setting is the physical environment: nature, or some very safe-feeling and quiet place, using headphones to block out ambient sound.

Sitter: Your Psychedelic Safari Guide

RLM: What is the sitter?

JE: Well, I sometimes lose some of my hipper, younger friends when I say you should take it with a guide. A guide is someone who knows the terrain, who's been there a number of times, who is not disturbed by a little difficulty. The reason for having a guide is the same reason you start with a guide when scuba diving or learning to fly a plane. The image that makes the most sense to me is of a safari guide, say in Africa. He doesn't see the animals for you, but he may say, "You see that rhinoceros that's running toward us? If I were you I would stand behind a tree." Or, he may say, "That little patch of sand in front, to your right? That's actually quicksand. You might want to walk around that."

So a guide or coach seems to be invaluable if you are taking your own experience seriously and you're interested in using the materials the way they've been used in a sacred way in every culture we know of that had access to it.

Substance: "What" and "How Much"?

RLM: What do you mean when you say the "substance"?

JE: What you take matters. There is an enormous list of psychedelic substances: mushrooms, peyote, and mescaline, all of which have the same basic set of experiences available. The biggest difference is a psilocybin (mushroom) experience lasts six to eight hours and LSD lasts usually eight to twelve hours. LSD is the one I know the best.

There are other psychedelic families, including the one that is most exciting to people these days, called ayahuasca. Ayahuasca is really two plants combined together, and they have a much different, much more physical expression, and it takes you to a very different part of the radio dial of consciousness.

What you take matters, and how much you take matters enormously. If you take too much of anything—that includes aspirin and peanut butter—you will get ill. With psychedelics, that "too much" is of two sorts. One is you really won't know where you are, and you can become disorganized and more frightened. Two—and for me this is equally important—you really won't remember the useful or beneficial parts. You'll simply have had an experience that you have no remembrance of. Some people take too much to prove how macho they are, and that's just a waste of everyone's time. If you take a small dose, obviously you'll have less of an experience. The purpose of the guide is so you don't make a mistake about what's correct for your body and your intention.

RLM: What is an appropriate dose if one wants to do inner-space work—one wants to explore and learn about oneself? What is a substantial dose of LSD in micrograms?

JF: One hundred to 200 micrograms is the dose people have used historically when they are working psychotherapeutically. If you're working for spiritual experiences it's double that [200 to 400 micrograms]. For people who are alcoholics—and the alcoholism research with LSD is excellent—it is usually necessary to take a larger dose, because they are used to alcohol, and it's stifling their own altered state inside themselves. Again, the guide turns out to be invaluable. Giving dosage numbers over the air, given how different people are, is simply not the correct service.

RLM: Understood. But what you're saying across the board, in terms of the normal curve, is that 300 to 400 micrograms is more of a spiritual dose, and 100 to 200 micrograms is more a dose for psychotherapeutic inner work.

JF: Right, psychotherapeutic inner work, where again, you need someone else with you. And if you're going for the higher doses, a guide is an absolute necessity if you wish to discover what it is that the classical mystics are talking about.

RLM: Is a higher dose 500, 600, 700 micrograms, or more?

JF: No, it's 300 to 400 micrograms.

RLM: I see. What happens when you get above 400 micrograms?

JF: My recommendation is: **don't**. You bring back too little and you risk too much.

Session: The Duration of Mind Alteration

RLM: What is meant by the "Session," Jim?

JF: A session is the hours when the substance is affecting you. We're talking about a substance in millionths of a gram. It actually leaves the body in about 1.5 hours, so most everything that goes on is within your own body and within your own body chemistry. But this is a full day or full night of events, and therefore you need to plan for that entire time.

Remember we need to reiterate—both my personal taste and my publisher's taste is to remind you—these are illegal substances, and that affects all these things. These are illegal substances, and people are imprisoned for far longer than anybody thinks is sane for both using and distributing. Therefore, this is not to suggest that anybody should use these, because they are illegal. But a bit like sex, you're probably going to be interested in it, so you might as well understand it. If you go ahead and do it, you might as well do it with some good sense to prevent illness, disease, and so forth.

With that caveat, this is only for people who have some understanding of what I'm talking about from their prior experience. We are looking at the ways to make things safe. What are the ways that lead to what is called a learning experience? Because we're not just talking about a single experience, like a roller coaster. A recent article pointed out that people who took psilocybin for spiritual purposes at Johns Hopkins University were still, fourteen months later, what they called "more open to the creative" and "more open to relationships"—basically a healthier person as well as psychology can measure.*

RLM: I can feel my blood starting to boil when you talk about that study, Jim. I'm thinking about fifty years of government suppression of these psychedelic medicines. Here we have one psychedelic medicine, which the people took one time, and a year later they're still having positive effects. How many medicines do we have in our entire pharmacopeia that you can take one time and a year later you're still feeling positive effects?

Basically, in the pharmaceutical industry you sign up for an annuity, right? You're going to be taking the medication daily and paying for it for the rest of your life. On the other hand we have a psychedelic medicine people can take one time, and a full year later they're still feeling measurable positive effects. However, no one can buy this new medicine right now. No one can get it legally. Your doctor can't prescribe it to you—there's nowhere you can get it legally in the United States. Isn't that correct?

JF: Let me add, Richard, a wonderful bit of film footage I saw recently about someone who took LSD once forty years ago, who was a serious, heavy-duty alcoholic—losing his job, his marriage was falling apart, life was terrible, and he was totally addicted. He took LSD once in a safe, secure, therapeutic setting, and forty years later, the filmmaker asks if he's had alcohol since then. He said, "Oh no, not a drop." The filmmaker then says something about willpower, and the man laughs and says, "No. No interest."

The change is about learning—about worldview and changing the way you see things. We really need to begin to let go of the medical model. As you were saying, the medical model says, "Pill in, body

---

*R. R. Griffiths et al., "Psilocybin Occasioned Mystical-type Experiences: Immediate and Persisting Dose-related Effects," *Psychopharmacology* 218, no. 4 (2011): 649–65. (See chapter 3.)

changes. Pill out, body back to normal. Needs more pills for next cycle." Psychedelics are really more like discovery. You only have to go to Europe once to find out that the world is much larger than the United States. You don't have to keep going back every week to be reminded.

RLM: Yes, the psychedelic medicine finds the atherosclerosis of the spirit and cleans it out. It's like a spiritual Roto-Rooter, and it gets all the junk out of us and clears us up.

JF: Right—one wants to see something that relaxes the hardening of the attitudes.

Life Group: Supportive Community

RLM: Jim Fadiman is all about safety. I totally support that—I'm all about safety myself. The sixth thing on your list of the six essential things to know for a safe psychedelic journey is the life group after. Tell us about what that means psychologically. Tell us about the life group that you come into after you've had this psychedelic experience.

JF: Remember that for over 80 percent of people in one study, taking a psychedelic was the most important experience of their life. Basically, the lifegroup is seen if you had this kind of transformative experience and you come back home to your family, and they say, "Isn't that wonderful! We really are delighted that you also now understand what we've known," or if you come back to your family and friends and they say, "That's nonsense. You're not supposed to know about God. There are books for that. You're always supposed to go to some other authority to ask their opinion," or even worse if they say, "This is craziness, and we're not sure that you should be allowed to go to work!"

We're talking about what kind of worldview you are in. Fortunately, knowing a lot about your sphere of radio influence, there's not much of a problem in this part of California, because so many people have already had these kinds of experiences and are basically aware that the material world simply can't be all there is. No culture but ours has ever made that materialistic assumption, and as we all know, we got it wrong. The world is being loused up by people who have forgotten that the interconnectedness of all things turns out to be very important.

•••

In this chapter we have heard reports of the scientific findings of four leading scientists—from the United States, England, and Czechoslovakia—representing over 160 years of combined research experience. What they have discovered is that psychedelic medicines have huge potential for healing, creativity, and personal transformation. These medicines, when used properly, are safe with virtually no negative side effects. Keeping these medicines illegal is a cruel affront to the public who are being denied access to their curative and transformational powers.

TWO

MDMA

Heart Medicine

Substance: MDMA (3,4-methylenedioxymethamphetamine), a.k.a. Molly, ecstasy, X, E, XTC, Adam.

Schedule: I*

The psychoactive medicine 3,4-methylenedioxymethamphetamine (MDMA) is presently used primarily as a recreational drug—because it is illegal to use it for its most important purpose: psychotherapy. Effects include significantly increased empathy, mild euphoria, personal insight, and heightened sensations including sexual sensations. When taken by mouth, effects begin after thirty to forty minutes and last two to four hours.

MDMA increases the release and slows the reuptake of the neurotransmitters serotonin, dopamine, and norepinephrine in parts of the brain.

MDMA was first synthesized in 1912. It was used to improve psychotherapy beginning in the 1970s and became popular as a street drug in the 1980s. In 2014 up to 29 million people between the ages of fifteen and sixty-four used ecstasy.

---

*No recognized medical use and high potential for abuse.

MDMA is generally illegal in most countries. Researchers are investigating whether a few low doses of MDMA may assist in treating severe, treatment-resistant post-traumatic stress disorder. In November 2016, Phase III clinical trials for PTSD were approved by the United States Food and Drug Administration to assess effectiveness and safety.

A Cherubic Cheerleader for Psychedelic Research

Our first interviewee, Rick Doblin, PhD, is by far the world's foremost—and, if I may add, cherubic—cheerleader for psychedelic research. When I met him in 1985 at Esalen, he was full of enthusiasm for his dream. He planned on going to Harvard, getting a PhD, and then founding a pharmaceutical company that would fund research around the world into psychedelics. He accomplished all of these things and more. His insights into MDMA in the following interview are invaluable.

Drawing a Map from "X" to Rx
Rick Doblin, PhD
March 5, 2013 (with excerpts from August 18, 2015)

RICK DOBLIN, PHD, is the founder and executive director of the Multidisciplinary Association for Psychedelic Studies (MAPS). He received his doctorate in public policy from Harvard's Kennedy School of Government, where he wrote his dissertation on the regulation of the medical uses of psychedelics and marijuana. His professional goal is to help develop legal contexts for the beneficial uses of psychedelics and marijuana, primarily as prescription medicines but also for personal growth for otherwise healthy people, and eventually to become a legally licensed psychedelic therapist.

The Long Road to the Pentagon

RLM: Rick, welcome to *Mind, Body, Health & Politics.*

Rick Doblin, PhD (RD): Richard, it's a pleasure.

RLM: How are you?

RD: Really good. Super excited actually. On Monday I'm going to an appointment at the Pentagon to meet various Department of Defense officials, and later that afternoon I'm going to the Senate. We're proposing a demonstration project with active-duty military with post-traumatic stress disorder [PTSD], where we would train the therapists, they would provide the active-duty military, and we would do MDMA-assisted psychotherapy.

They would have their own independent raters evaluating the patients, and we hope they can fund additional studies if they can see it work. If we get permission for this first study, it would be a tiny little nonprofit, MAPS, giving a grant to the Department of Defense.*

Coming of Age in a Time of Change

RLM: Let us back up just a little bit. Over twenty-five years ago, Dr. Rick Doblin—well, he wasn't *Dr.* Rick Doblin when we first met in the early 1980s at the Esalen Institute—started MAPS, the Multidisciplinary Association for Psychedelic Studies, which supports pioneering, groundbreaking research on the psychoactive substances MDMA, ayahuasca, DMT, ibogaine, ketamine, LSD, mescaline, peyote, psilocybin, and salvia divinorum.

Research into these substances has been virtually nonexistent and has been suppressed by the United States government for the last

---

*Greg Miller, "A Psychedelic-Science Advocate Takes His Case to the Pentagon," WIRED.com, May 2013, https://www.wired.com/2013/05/doblin/ (accessed April 30, 2017).

fifty years. We're going to find out from Rick how he managed to start MAPS in the face of this governmental and political suppression. Why did you start MAPS over twenty-five years ago?

RD: Let's go back a little bit further. In 1972, when I was eighteen years old, I had my first experiences with LSD. I had been educated to believe one dose of LSD made you permanently crazy, and I was fearful of these drugs, but I also had a lot of questions about the accuracy of the information I was being taught. I read *One Flew Over the Cuckoo's Nest*, by Ken Kesey, and a friend of mine told me after I'd read it that Kesey wrote part of it under the influence of LSD. I'm thinking, "That can't be possible—this is such a fantastic book." When I tried LSD, I felt like it started doing what my bar mitzvah was supposed to do.

RLM: Turned you into a man?

RD: Yeah, it was an existential challenge—it was opening up my emotions. I felt something fundamentally deep and profound was impacted. For a lot of us, traditional rituals, religious services, and rites of passage are more intellectual than deep and profound. So I woke up to the incredible value of psychedelics, just as the backlash from the sixties was coming into full power.

RLM: 1972—Nixon got elected.

RD: It was disheartening to see the potential of these [now illegal] substances. I'd also been aware of the Holocaust—born in 1953, growing up Jewish—and of how people project outward, disown their shadow, and put it on others. I felt the problems of survival had a lot to do with psychological factors. The technological advancement we've enjoyed through the incredible development of the mind—just miraculous technology—has outstripped our emotional and spiritual capabilities to handle it wisely. So we have global warming, we have the threat of nuclear weapons, and all sorts of environmental devastation. I felt that—both for me as an individual and for society—we needed to become more balanced with the emotional-spiritual side of ourselves.

Also, I had a very difficult time with the LSD and went to the guidance counselor at my college, New College in Sarasota, Florida, and he gave me a manuscript copy of *Realms of the Human Unconscious* by Stanislav Grof, which was inspiring. It wasn't philosophy. It wasn't basic science. It was therapy. It focused on how to actually help people, in a way, as reality testing. So I decided to devote myself to psychedelic research, spirituality, values, and reality testing of therapy. But everything was shut down, and I felt like I didn't have any opportunities. I needed to work on myself more so that I would be capable of handling all of these energies. Then ten years later, in 1982, I went back to school and was able to do my first semester back, at Esalen, during a month-long workshop with Stanislav and Christina Grof. During that time, somebody came by and started talking about MDMA, which was legal at the time.

A New Tool for Self-Discovery

RLM: Tell us what MDMA stands for please.

RD: MDMA is methylenedioxymethamphetamine, more popularly known as ecstasy, or Molly. It's a semisynthetic drug, so it is not found in nature by itself in that form, but it comes from sassafras—safrole—and is somewhat modified chemically. It is gentler than the classic psychedelics. Some people have tried to give it other names, like entactogen or empathogen, because you don't get the classic visual impacts on your train of thought—the flow, or emergence, of the unconscious—that happens under classic psychedelics or in dream states. MDMA is gentler than that, and it opens up emotional capabilities. It reduces fear and anxiety. It promotes a sense of self-acceptance and peace, and it can be used in many different ways.

I learned there was a tradition of therapists and psychiatrists continuing to work with substances, particularly MDMA, in a quiet, underground way. But some people who had used it therapeutically realized there was a major market for other uses, so they turned it into ecstasy, which started being sold in recreational contexts, attracting the attention of the government. It felt like I had a chance to do history all over again in that I had learned about MDMA before the crackdown, but it was clear that the crackdown was coming; this was the rise of Nancy Reagan's "Just Say No" and the drug war in full flower.

I felt like we needed to organize and prepare for the crackdown, so I had an incredible opportunity to work with psychiatrists and psychologists, and I also worked with Robert Muller, who was the assistant secretary general of the United Nations. He'd written a book, *New Genesis: Shaping a Global Spirituality,* about how the United Nations exists to help mediate conflicts between countries, but how many conflicts go deeper, to religious conflicts. They felt we needed a mystical sense that people could come together with unity while still appreciating all the differences and uniqueness of religions. He realized psychedelics could be a tool in studying religion and spirituality, and so he decided to help me bring back psychedelic research.

RLM: This was before MDMA was made illegal, in the early '80s.

RD: I worked with Brother David Steindl-Rast, and Rabbi Zalman Schachter, and others who were lifelong Zen meditators. They were willing to use MDMA in small, roughly half-doses in meditation, which they found could facilitate deeper learning. Students could practice on their own, making progress in ways that they had not been able to do before.

The DEA Schedules MDMA

RD: Starting in 1984, the Drug Enforcement Administration [DEA] finally decided to criminalize MDMA. When they criminalize a substance, they have to file something in the Federal Register, and then there are thirty days to file an appeal. We were prepared for that. We'd even done a safety study in around thirty-two people on Stinson Beach for the first study ever of MDMA, which we kept quiet. Just looking at blood pressure and heart rate and various other . . .

RLM: That's the study that Dr. Jack Downing was involved with?

RD: Yes, that was the first study ever on MDMA.

RLM: Yes, I remember that. My therapist Robert Kantor gave me MDMA as part of my therapy in 1982 and 1983, while it was still legal. And Leo Zeff, PhD, aka the Secret Chief, whom I think you knew . . .

RD: He was in charge of handing out the MDMA at the experiment.

RLM: Leo lived four doors away from me in Kensington, California, at the time, so I was a regular subject of his.

RD: Lucky.

RLM: Very lucky.

RD: So we completely took the DEA by surprise. They had become aware of ecstasy, but the code name for MDMA was Adam when it was used in these therapeutic settings, and about half a million doses had been distributed and used since the mid '70s to the early '80s, and the DEA had no knowledge of that. There were no problems from it. It didn't come to public attention—so they just thought they were criminalizing a recreational drug, and they were shocked when I walked in the door in Washington and handed them a petition with pro bono legal representation from a major DC law firm, and testimony from Harvard Medical School psychiatrist Lester Grinspoon and George Greer and others who had experience with MDMA and were willing to say, in public, that they thought that it should remain available to psychiatrists and therapists.

We were able to have what's called an administrative law judge hearing in front of a DEA administrative law judge, arguing it was premature to criminalize it, and that it should remain available as a therapeutic tool. To our astonishment and to my great faith now in parts of the American political system, we won the lawsuit. The judge recommended that MDMA be made illegal for recreational use but that it remain available legally for therapeutic use. These administrative law judges make recommendations to the head of the agency that they're working in. So this went to the administrator of the DEA who decided that this was a recommendation that he didn't want to accept, and he rejected the recommendation. That was heartbreaking for us—we won the lawsuit and then the DEA rejected the recommendations.

Then we decided to sue in the appeals courts, and we won several times, but eventually the DEA was able to satisfy the court that they had a set of criteria that would criminalize MDMA completely, and that would be that.

How to Start
a Psychedelic Pharmaceutical Company
The Only Way Is through FDA

RLM: You still had not started MAPS at that point.

RD: Right. For a long time we had an international strategy to try to start research everywhere else in the world, because we were blocked in the United States. Once it became clear that the United States could manipulate things around the world, we had to go back and start inside the United States with the Food and Drug Administration [FDA]. It became clear that the only way to bring it back was not through lawsuits that we had won but then lost, but through the FDA. At the time I had this naive hope, because there were hundreds of thousands—eventually millions—of people using MDMA, and I thought that if they all just donated a dollar or two then we would have the funds necessary to do the research. In 1986 I started MAPS as a nonprofit pharmaceutical company trying to develop psychedelics and marijuana into FDA-approved prescription medicines.

RLM: So, in effect, you formed a pharmaceutical company.

RD: Yes, I wasn't quite aware of it at the time, but there had never been a nonprofit development of a drug. That changed in 2000. The first example of a successful nonprofit drug development was the abortion pill, Mifepristone, produced by the Population Council with funding by the Rockefeller family, Warren Buffett, who donated over $5 million to it, the Pritzker family, and others. They teamed up and took a drug that was highly controversial and that pharmaceutical companies would not research because their other products would be boycotted, and brought it to market. The FDA was willing to work with a nonprofit organization, and that was a success.

I didn't know that it had never been done when I started MAPS, but I felt that it could be done and should be done and that it was the only way forward. I believed in science. I really did believe in the scientific process, and I respected the work that was done by the FDA to evaluate drugs. The genesis of MAPS was trying to gather together all the people that were having these profound personal experiences that were beneficial to them and to say, let's all put our resources together and try to fund studies that will satisfy the skeptics and critics and the regulators at the FDA.

The Mission to Legalize MDMA as Prescription Medicine

RLM: And your mission . . .

RD: Primarily, it was to develop MDMA into a prescription medicine. But of course I broadened it to all psychedelics and marijuana. MAPS is also chartered to look at non-drug techniques as well, like holotropic breathwork, hyperventilation, meditation, and spirituality. MAPS can actually do a large number of things consistent with our articles of incorporation, but the core element was to work politically and scientifically. Then I was an undergraduate, wanting to become a PhD in clinical psychology in order to do psychotherapy-outcome research with MDMA and LSD—to show that it really was helpful.

In 1987, when I graduated, I tried to get into various clinical psychology PhD programs, telling them I was interested in doing MDMA research, which was still illegal. The crackdown that began in the mid '60s was complete by the early '70s. By the mid '80s, research was still squashed and researchers were locked out of the laboratories. You couldn't do any science.

It was frustrating. So I sat down and I thought about it, and I realized that I wanted to do the science, but the politics were in the way. And I had this insight: maybe I should just switch my focus and study the politics.

I had read an interview in *Harper's Magazine* with a fellow named Mark Kleiman and several others who were drug-policy experts, and they mentioned the lawsuit that I had been involved in. I decided to call up Mark Kleiman, who turned out to be a professor at the Kennedy School of Government at Harvard. I told him my situation—that I only had one class in politics, and that was a class about suing the DEA—everything else was in psychology. But I asked him if he would be my mentor, and he said he would and he encouraged me to apply. So I ended up getting a master's and a PhD from the Kennedy School of Government at Harvard with my dissertation focused on regulation of the medical use of psychedelics and marijuana.

RLM: Meanwhile, you had already started MAPS in the mid '80s. You were already starting to get donations. Had you already funded any research by then?

RD: No, since all the research was still blocked.

Overcoming the Global Suppression of Research

RLM: When you say research on psychedelic materials was squashed, what immediately comes to mind is that trip, to Israel, I had the good fortune of joining you on. We consulted with Israeli officials about the possibility of using MDMA with their PTSD patients, because so many Israeli citizens there had witnessed horrific events during the Intifada. We were told by the government of Israel that they would love to do the MAPS research study but they couldn't, because if they did the research, the United States government would sanction them. That was the first time in my life I came face-to-face with how the United States government squashes research around the planet. Now is that still the case? Where are we now with regard to other countries doing psychedelic medicine research?

RD: That was so disheartening. It really was. We had to start MDMA–PTSD research in the United States before we could get started in Israel, because it is so dependent on the security of the United States. Once we started it in the United States, however, they were still nervous, until we began a second study at Harvard Medical School with MDMA for cancer patients with anxiety. That helped the Israelis realize that they weren't going to get any pressure from the United States for doing things that were already happening in the United States.

We have a study at the largest mental hospital in Israel with the former chief psychiatrist of the Israel Defense Forces as the principal investigator. Interestingly enough, one of the meetings that we had, when you and I were in Israel, was with the Israeli antidrug authority; so not only did we have to get approval from the Ministry of Health, we had to get approval from the antidrug authority. Just recently the Israeli government eliminated the antidrug authority—defunded it completely—so we're seeing a worldwide recognition that prohibition has gone too far and that one of the consequences of prohibition was to restrict research of beneficial uses of medicines that were prohibited, such as marijuana, MDMA, and LSD. Now that the zeal for prohibition is declining, and we're seeing movements toward the legalization of marijuana and an opposition to mass incarceration, we are able to do research with MDMA in almost any country in the world. It looks like next week I'll be going to Israel, and we are starting our MDMA–PTSD study there, in association with the Ministry of Health in the Israel Defense Forces.

RLM: What is it, ten years later from our trip to Israel?

RD: Yes.

RLM: But you persist. You persist, Rick, and it is so wonderful that you continue to persevere.

MAPS: The Intersection of Politics, Science, and Psychedelics

RLM: It is over twenty-five years from when you started MAPS in 1985. Tell us about the research that MAPS is sponsoring in these various psychedelic medicines that I listed.

RD: The good news is that there is now more psychedelic research taking place around the world than at any time in the last forty years. We're basically combining science, politics, and psychedelics. We've realized that because these drugs and their users are stigmatized we have to be very strategic about which drug and which patient population we start doing the studies with. Our resources are limited, and we want to do work that will have the biggest appeal to the American public.

I got my master's from 1988–1990, and I got a Presidential Management Fellowship for people who want careers in the federal government and applied for a job at the FDA. In 1990 the group at the FDA with the authority to regulate psychedelics and marijuana switched to a new group, and they wanted to put science before politics. That's where things really started.

Two Phases Down,
One More to Approval

RD: It's been almost twenty-three years since then. We started from what are called Phase I studies—working in a healthy population to evaluate what the drug does—to get a sense of the risk and to get a sense of the potential patients. Phase II is where you can start working with patients, and Phase III are the large-scale, definitive studies.

We're in the middle of the Phase II stage all over the world—working with patients. Of the patients we've chosen—again for these political reasons—the first are those with PTSD. People are very sympathetic to those who have been victimized: those who have survived childhood sexual abuse, adult rape and assault, or particularly now veterans and soldiers with PTSD from the wars in Iraq and Afghanistan; or those in Israel from wars and terrorism, all over the world.

Our primary focus is MDMA, because it's a gentler psychedelic than the rest. We've actually heard from a lot of people who had difficult psychedelic trips with LSD or psilocybin or mescaline during the '60s or '70s—during their youth—who have been unable to work through them, and when they smoke marijuana it brings it back. A fair number of people I know don't use marijuana because it brings back difficult psychedelic trips from the past; and we worked with some of these people and have found that MDMA can help them integrate these difficult psychedelic experiences.

I think MDMA will be the first drug that will be integrated into our culture, and I think PTSD is likely to be the first clinical indication, and we're seeing lots of support. That's why we're being invited to go to the Pentagon to present this proposal. Combining these two directions—both the politics of drug regulation and also psychotherapy—has led me to conclude that MDMA has an excellent chance of making it through the regulatory system.

Maximizing Benefits and Minimizing Risks of MDMA-Assisted Therapy

The Session: How Often Is Too Often?

RLM: Is there a negative effect of frequent use of MDMA, and what is frequent use?

RD: Every drug has its risks, and MDMA is not a magical drug that has no risks. Our model is a male/female co therapist team in a therapeutic setting. It's roughly a 3.5-month treatment process, and there are initially three weekly, non-medicine, ninety-minute sessions to build the therapeutic alliance between the therapist and the patients—to come to understand the history of each one's trauma and of how each patient has reacted.

Then there is an MDMA session, which starts at around 10 a.m. and goes to 6 p.m.—an eight-hour session. Then patients spend the night in the treatment center. The MDMA sessions are then followed by a non-medicine therapy session the next day, after which the patients receive phone calls every day for a week, followed by weekly non-medicine psychotherapy for a month.

The MDMA sessions in our therapeutic setting are three to five weeks apart. In our first study, we did a series of very complicated and expensive neurocognitive studies, because the claim has been that MDMA will reduce serotonin if it's done too frequently or at too-high doses, and then people will supposedly have cognitive deficiencies. We tested that and found no evidence at all. In our therapeutic setting, with pure MDMA spaced out once a month—three times—there's no evidence that it's harmful.

Now, if people were to do it every other day, I think that would be too frequent. I have seen some people that have done it too frequently, and they get the opposite of what they were looking for. They're looking for a heightened emotionality, deeper feelings of peace and love; but when you just continue to do it too frequently you kind of get muted in your emotions. You become much more washed out and drained.

RLM: On the other hand, Rick, I've had patients—couples—who have done it once a week, every single week for up to a year, and they report very beneficial effects.

RD: Yeah. There is so much individual variability.

RLM: I see.

Integrating the Experience

RD: In terms of frequency, the key part is for me is whether the patient integrated what happened before. So if you're just looking for the experience itself and not thinking about what you bring back from it, and how you adjust and grow in your daily non-drug life . . .

RLM: Non-medicine life, shall we say?

RD: Yeah, I think that's a healthy way to say, "Okay, I'm going to have this experience. It's for the experience itself, but it's also for what I bring back from it—what I've learned from it." And then once you've integrated it, then I think you're ready if you want to do it again.

RLM: That's true of all the psychedelic medicines, isn't it? That the key is bringing the information back over the line, into daily life?

RD: Yeah, that's exactly right.

RLM: Whether it's ayahuasca, LSD, ibogaine—with all of the psychedelics—there's an opportunity for gigantic learning; but then we are challenged to bring that gigantic learning right back into, quote, "the real world."

RD: Yeah. These are tools to help enhance our non-drug life. This is a voyage that you take—like a vacation you take—but you come back to your life, and then hopefully you feel refreshed and rejuvenated. I think there's something to the serotonin changes that government-funded researchers have highlighted or exaggerated. But in the therapeutic doses that we use, and for many people using even larger doses in recreational settings, they don't see these problems.

Not Too Much, Not Too Little: Finding a "Goldilocks" Dose

RLM: What is the therapeutic dose that you've been using with MDMA?

RD: We use 125 milligrams, and then between 1.5 and 2.5 hours later we administer a supplemental dose of half the initial dose.

RLM: And what is considered a large dose?

RD: Sometimes people outside of clinical settings will take two pills—or 250 milligrams—or sometimes even more.

RLM: Do we have any negative effects on record of people taking very large doses and something not good happening to them?

RD: There are rare instances, yes, of people in recreational settings that take MDMA and are engaged in vigorous dancing while not drinking adequate fluids, and they'll overheat—hyperthermia.

RLM: Thus, we have artifacts affecting results because it's not the medicine that causes negative effects, rather it is taking the medicine in what Jim Fadiman would say is the improper setting, one which itself causes hyperthermia—such as taking hot baths or other factors—which the MDMA exacerbates.

RD: MDMA has pharmacologically built-in safeguards against abuse. The classic addictive drug is one that you take a lot and you build up a tolerance to it, and so then you just up the dose. Before you know it, you're taking these huge doses and you're dependent on the drugs. With MDMA, if you take it very frequently and lose the feeling—the depth of it—you try to take a higher dose, but it doesn't work. You get more of the amphetamine, more of the speedy part of it, but not the peaceful part of it. It doesn't encourage the traditional pattern of an addictive drug with tolerance and ever-larger doses.

RLM: I read a study indicating that some people actually do better on a smaller dose. What can you tell us about MDMA dosage and boosters?

RD: We've tried that, and that hasn't worked. Part of my dissertation was about how to do double-blind studies with drugs like MDMA, where it's pretty easy to tell if you've got an inactive placebo or the full dose. The approach I arrived at after a lot of thought was a "dose–response," meaning everybody knows they're going to get MDMA, but they don't know what the dose will be. If you show a dose–response relationship, then that would be sufficient. The low doses in the neighborhood of 25 to 30 milligrams seem to have had an antitherapeutic effect. People get activated, but they don't get the peacefulness—the reduction of fear—so they're actually confronting their negative emotions or their trauma without the support that they would need. So that's antitherapeutic. And when you start getting higher and higher, we discovered something absolutely surprising, which is that the 75 milligram dose is doing remarkably well, to where the responses are really indistinguishable from full doses.

Supplementing MDMA to Reduce Fatigue

RLM: I want to read to you an email I got from a psychiatrist friend, Dr. Bruce Africa. He says:

> Please let Rick Doblin know that I have immensely appreciated his efforts in bringing intelligent, rational thought to the subject of psychedelic drugs and their place in society. But I also have a question about the negative effects, and if there are side effects, such as fatigue? What can be taken along with the MDMA, in advance, in order to ameliorate this fatigue? And what are the other negative effects you might mention?

RD: The first thing to say is that many people, myself included, feel exhausted the day after taking MDMA. In our therapy, we take advantage of that as a reason to talk about this as a two-day experience, where the second day is for people to rest, reflect, and integrate what happened the first day. When we do our therapy, people are required to spend the night in the treatment center. They can have a significant other come and spend the night if they want, and then the next day they have a leisurely morning. They have several hours of non-drug integration of psychotherapy. They can't drive home—somebody else has to come take them home—and they're encouraged to rest.

Then we call them every day on the phone for the first week. This exhaustion, when there is such a rush in our modern world, is a rather novel occurrence for a lot of people, and so we've woven that into the therapy. Also, to answer your question: we are trying to figure out what MDMA does by itself, so we don't administer any substances, before or after, to help ease this exhaustion or to increase the depth of the experience. However, people have talked about 5-HTP, which is a serotonin precursor that can be taken either before and/or after: before to try to make the experience deeper and after to try to recover more quickly from the exhaustion.

RLM: I've heard reports that 5-HTP has been helpful, and it's an over-the-counter medicine.

RD: Yeah. It's just a serotonin precursor, and it's something that a lot of people say does help with the exhaustion.

RLM: What about tyrosine, lysine, tryptophan? Any report on those?

RD: No, you really need to go to Erowid.org, where there are all sorts of personal accounts of people that have combined various things with MDMA for different purposes. Even though there is massive experience from tens of millions having done MDMA, all of that has taken place outside of the experimental context, so we don't have any scientific information about it. When we negotiate with the FDA or the European Medicines Agency we've been instructed to just assume we know nothing and then start from the beginning—the ground up, so to speak. We needed to see how strong the side effects actually were, and it turns out in our model it's not much of a problem. People are more exhausted when they take it at night during a party and then go do stuff the next day and don't eat or drink properly. We find that people welcome the time-out the next day to reflect, and it is an integral part of our treatment. There is a lot to learn in regard to combinations, but we don't have any direct information.

One of the concerns that was expressed thirty years ago about MDMA was that one dose causes permanent brain damage—that people would be suffering significant and severe functional consequences. But nobody was at the time, and so they reasoned that this is the kind of thing that's going to show up over time: "We can't see it right now, but as people age they're going to start showing all these symptoms. Their brains will decline, and the symptoms that are covered up by redundancy in the brain are going to be showing up later." Now we have people that have aged, and we don't see these symptoms. That whole time-bomb theory of MDMA neurotoxicity has been discredited.

RLM: It's certainly been discredited in my life. My therapist, Dr. Robert Kantor, gave MDMA to me during our sessions in the early '80s—I know I've taken it over a hundred times—and while I do misplace my keys and glasses quite often, I think I'm still able to talk to you coherently.

Evidence of Safety in Clinical Setting

RLM: You said tens of millions of people have taken MDMA. We do not have reports coming in from all over the United States, as we did with cocaine and heroin, about emergency room admittances from

MDMA overdoses. Tens of millions of people use this medicine with very few negative effects. We humans know when a substance is dangerous. I mean, if you ingest a bit of rat poison, or a little tiny bit of arsenic, or a little tiny bit of something that gives you the runs, and you know it immediately.

When you have something that's ingested by the public for ten, twenty, thirty, or fifty years with no negative results—that counts as part of science, is referred to as anecdotal evidence over time, and deserves to be taken very seriously. In my work at Wilbur Hot Springs, where people have been taking the medicinal waters for 150 years, there has never been one complaint to a health department. That record means a great deal, because when people sit in water, some of it goes in their mouths and other bodily orifices. If there's something in the water that will make them sick, it would eventually get reported and certainly we would be aware of the danger after ten, twenty, or thirty years, let alone 150 years. Anecdotal evidence over 150 years tells us this Wilbur Springs medicinal water has no unwanted complications, aka harmful side effects. How does this evidence of tens of millions of people safely using this MDMA medicine—along with tens of millions of people using marijuana and LSD—fail to positively affect the public, the psychiatric profession, and the law-making politicians? Does this massive amount of use without harm not influence in any way how the government acts?

RD: Well, it doesn't influence it directly. To make drugs into medicine you need data from FDA-approved studies. But it does make the FDA comfortable about MDMA or marijuana in ways that they're not comfortable about any other drug ever approved, because when pharmaceutical companies try to get a drug through, at the most there will be ten thousand subjects. There are usually several thousand or even several hundred subjects studied to get a drug approved as a medicine.

Once the drugs are released into the market, then you have the one-in-one-hundred-thousand side effect or the one-in-a-million side effect. That's where you see a lot of drugs withdrawn from the market—*after* it seemed to the FDA and the pharmaceutical industry that they were sufficiently safe. With MDMA and these substances that have been used by tens of millions of people, we know the one-in-a-million side effects: we know that sometimes people can overheat and die when they're dancing all night without adequate fluid replacement. We know that sometimes people can die from taking MDMA and drinking too much water, causing hyponatremia.

"Ecstasy" Off the Street

RLM: Is there a difference between MDMA and ecstasy?

RD: There shouldn't be. Ecstasy, when it originally came out, was another name for MDMA, but now I almost never use the word *ecstasy* to describe what we're doing because it's impure. Recent studies have shown that most drugs sold as ecstasy or Molly are not pure MDMA—you usually get MDMA mixed with stuff or no MDMA at all. We had the eighth employee at Microsoft, Bob Wallace, donate about $100,000 for an ecstasy pill-testing program in order to protect and give some knowledge to the people who were purchasing it illegally. It turned out that over half of the samples had no MDMA in them at all, and there were all sorts of adulterants—methamphetamine, ketamine, caffeine. Ecstasy was a term meant to refer to MDMA, but now it's very difficult to say what's really in it.

RLM: Understood. So it's the difference between a real pharmaceutical-grade chemical and something off the street, where you have no idea what it is.

RD: Exactly. It's hard to say what the risks of pure MDMA are, but there have been over 1,100 people that have taken MDMA in a controlled, therapeutic, clinical research setting without any reported lasting negative consequences. Most of these people are healthy volunteers, not patients.

Early Treatments:
End-of-Life Suffering, PTSD, and Addiction

The Tremendous Need for End-of-Life Care

RLM: I just got a letter here that I want to read to you, Rick. This man writes in and says:

> I have a sister, sixty years old, who was diagnosed with stage 3.5 primary peritoneal cancer three years ago. She underwent debulking surgery, and then extensive chemo treatments for six months afterward. She coped well with the surgery and the chemo, and the cancer is still in remission. But she is miserable and suicidal. Her husband of forty years is beside himself with what to do.
>
> She has undergone electroconvulsive therapy and has rejected every medication she has been given from benzodiazepines to SSRIs to opiates. She's really losing her mind, and has already attempted suicide once, maybe more. She needs help, and I'm curious if you think there is anything you could suggest for her. I'm curious [this is where you come in, Rick] if there are any psychedelic-treatment studies you might be aware of that could be tried with her?

RD: Yes. There are two studies that are recruiting subjects, currently—one at NYU* and one at Johns Hopkins.† And so she could consider

---

*NYU Psilocybin Cancer Anxiety Study (this study is no longer accepting participants).
†Johns Hopkins Psilocybin Cancer Project (www.bpru.org/cancer-studies; note on website: The Johns Hopkins Psilocybin Research Project study team is pleased to report that enrollment for this study has now been completed).

applying to be a subject in both of those studies. I'm not sure if they would screen her out because of suicidality, but they might be willing to enroll her in the study.

RLM: I'm certainly willing to give it a shot. I'll send this gentleman an email with these two ideas.

RD: This work with end of life is very important as well. This is politically well chosen because everybody is going to be in that situation. Most people are more scared of dying than they are of drugs, so if you can show that psychedelic medicines can be helpful to them, they will listen. When people are facing anxiety from end of life, a lot of their anxiety has to do with their health status, and that change is independent of the therapy, so there is this other variable going on.

The other scientific challenge with the work we're doing—and with helping people be more peaceful about this existential "getting ready to die"—is that this kind of change is not so clearly mapped onto the current measures of anxiety that the FDA has used to approve drugs. We have to get these drugs approved by the FDA and the European Medicines Agency and then get insurance companies to cover it. So we still have a lot of challenges.

Measuring Benefits of MDMA for PTSD

RD: So there are some methodological challenges with this independent variable—the health status of the participants for the LSD and psilocybin work with end of life. It's easier to show therapeutic progress with MDMA for PTSD—the measure developed by the Department of Veteran Affairs [VA], called the Clinician Administered PTSD Scale [CAPS], does a great job of measuring PTSD symptoms.

There's so much need, it's incredible. We have over 250 people on the waiting list for the study with MDMA for post-traumatic stress in Charleston, and we have over fifty people on the waiting list for the

Boulder study, and we haven't even started the study yet.* Once the FDA evaluates the data, its head would be permitted to approve MDMA. We say we've noticed that MDMA reduces activity in the amygdala, or the fear-producing portion of the brain, and it increases activity in the frontal cortex, where we put things in association. It stimulates serotonin, dopamine, and norepinephrine, and it also releases oxytocin and prolactin—the hormones of nurturing and bonding. In contrast, PTSD reduces activity in the frontal cortex and increases activity in the amygdala.

There are only two drugs approved by the FDA for PTSD—Zoloft and Paxil—and they have marginal benefits. There is a large number of people that drop out of traditional non-drug psychotherapies— different estimates say 25 to 50 percent find traditional psychotherapy for PTSD to be retraumatizing rather than healing, because you have to relook at the trauma, and people are emotionally reactive or numb to it and avoid it.

At the same time, because of our foreign policy, we have a large number of veterans with PTSD that have failed to obtain relief from the currently available medications or psychotherapies that are being provided by the VA. Last year, the VA spent in the neighborhood of $6 billion just on disability payments to about thirty thousand veterans with PTSD. That's an annual figure that increases over time. These are young people, mostly, who are going to continue to grow and live for the next forty or fifty years. So there's an enormous moral debt that Americans feel toward these veterans. In addition, there is a growing awareness of the prevalence of childhood sexual abuse and adult rape and assault. People are realizing that there are way more people with PTSD from those causes than even from war-related PTSD. There was a terrific article in *Marie Claire*† about our MDMA and

*For information about completed, ongoing, and planned studies using MDMA, visit the MAPS "MDMA-Assisted Psychotherapy" page at www.maps.org/research/mdma.
†Kelley McMillan, "Is Ecstasy the Key to Treating Women with PTSD?" MarieClaire .com, August 17, 2015, www.marieclaire.com/health-fitness/news/a15553/mdma-ecstasy -drug-ptsd-treatment/ (accessed April 30, 2017).

PTSD research, and it highlighted some of the women subjects in our studies.

Treatment of Addiction Reveals the Mechanism of Recovery

RD: The third main area that we're trying to research is the treatment of addiction. It's a problem from a political point of view in that the addict is "the other." In terms of social change, it's not as powerful to develop treatments for the addict as working with people who are dying or with PTSD, but it offers this other opportunity to show that it's not about the drug.

The fundamental problem with our drug policy is that it ascribes good and bad qualities to drugs themselves—"this is a good drug, that's a bad drug"—when really it's the relationship that you have with the drug that determines the value of it and whether it's harmful or helpful. I think it was Paracelsus who said that the difference between a drug and a medicine—or a drug and a poison—is the dose. So by doing work with psychedelics with people who are struggling with dependence and addiction, we're able to demonstrate to people that psychedelics considered by the law to be drugs of abuse can help people overcome drug addiction in the proper circumstances. Bill W., who founded Alcoholics Anonymous [AA], used LSD in the 1950s and found it to be very helpful. It offers the two things that we know are important principles of Alcoholics Anonymous.

First is this idea of making amends and coming to terms with what you've done and overcoming denial. Psychedelics have this way of changing the mind in such a way that the things that people are repressing and denying and putting down come to the forefront. Sometimes people call it a "bad trip," or as we try to call it a "difficult trip," but you can learn from it. The second part of AA is this whole spiritual model and a higher power. So psychedelics in the treatment of addiction offer the opportunity for people to address and see what they have been trying to avoid and at the same time give them an opportunity for this unitive mystical experience of connection, from which they can draw strength to aid in their recovery.

Finding Common Ground with Psychedelics as well as Non-Drug Techniques

RD: There is also a series of studies being done on basic neuroscience and consciousness research asking what these drugs do in the brain. There is even a series of studies looking at the merging of religion and science in this forum in the sense of meditation, and this is extremely exciting for me. In the early '70s when the crackdown came, there was a large group of people who said, "We don't really need drugs—they're illegal. Let's explore non-drug alternatives." People have done that for the last forty years or so, and among the alternatives are yoga and meditation and various different techniques. People in their sixties are recognizing that they were inspired by their psychedelic experiences. Now there is a return to psychedelics—not in a frequent-use way, but in an inspirational way. We're working on starting research in Switzerland that would look at lifelong meditators who would be administered psilocybin in a meditation retreat.

Roland Griffiths at Johns Hopkins looked at whether people had mystical experiences. They were taking religiously inclined people—not just clergy, but people who have a religious or spiritual practice of some sort. An ideal experiment would be to take people in clergy from different religious traditions and have them go through whatever normal training they go through, and then also have a subgroup go through their normal training with the additional opportunity of psychedelic experiences. You could then compare how the people did with their peers in their own religion, and then you can look at the content of their experiences and compare a content analysis across all the different religions and look for the commonalities. I think we would find an awful lot of them. Eventually, people will be able to do this.

RLM: Fascinating.

RD: We believe it's not just about medical uses, it's about integrating psychedelics. In particular, it's about integrating the full range of consciousness into our mainstream society such that people have these profound senses of spiritual connection that I would equate to what astronauts who went to the moon felt when looking back at Earth.

RLM: Yes.

RD: If we can understand and appreciate our commonality, then we can all together face these incredible life-threatening changes happening to the planet, and we can appreciate differences rather than be scared of them.

RLM: Hear, hear, Rick. I think that's a perfect place to stop: to appreciate differences in each other rather than be afraid of them.

•••

My next interview on MDMA is with one of the first scientists to conduct government-approved psychobiological research on MDMA, Charlie Grob. I had the privilege of first meeting Charlie Grob at my home, in the early 1990s, during something called the "Friday night meetings," which were started by the Jungian analyst Dr. John Perry. These monthly meetings were an opportunity for researchers in the psychedelic community, from far and wide, to socialize and share ideas. Among many others, psychedelic pioneers Sasha and Anne Shulgin were regular attendees. It is a great honor to include this interview with Charlie Grob.

Pioneering Government-Approved Research
Charles Grob, MD
Excerpt from November 29, 2011

CHARLES S. GROB, MD, is director of the Division of Child and Adolescent Psychiatry at Harbor-UCLA Medical Center and Professor of Psychiatry and Pediatrics at the UCLA School of Medicine. In the early 1990s he conducted the first government-approved psychobiological research study of MDMA, and he was the principal investigator of an international research project in the Brazilian Amazon studying ayahuasca (see chapter 4). He has also completed an investigation of the safety and efficacy of psilocybin treatment in advanced-cancer patients with anxiety and published his findings in the January 2011 issue of the *Archives of General Psychiatry* (see chapter 3). He is the editor of *Hallucinogens: A Reader* (2002) and the coeditor (with Roger Walsh) of *Higher Wisdom: Eminent Elders Explore the Continuing Impact of Psychedelics* (State University of New York Press, 2005). He is a founding board member of the Heffter Research Institute.

The MDMA Neurotoxicity Scandal

RLM: You did the first government-approved psychological research study of MDMA. Please tell us about what you found.

Charles Grob, MD (CG): My initial involvement came after reading an article in the *Archives of General Psychiatry* in 1989 alleging that MDMA could cause permanent neurotoxic changes in the brains of human users. My colleagues and I felt there were some serious flaws in the article. The methodologies seemed somewhat questionable, so we published a letter to the editor critiquing the article's conclusions.

Shortly after, I received a call from Rick Doblin, whom I did not know at that time. Sasha Shulgin had shown him our letter to the editor that was published in the *Archives*. Rick contacted me and a colleague of mine when I was at UC Irvine and asked us if we were interested in submitting a protocol to the FDA on an application for MDMA. We wrote a protocol that would examine the effects of MDMA on a population of terminal cancer patients with anxiety, focusing on the anxiety and also pain.

The FDA examined our protocol and informed us that they could not approve a treatment study at that point because there had been no normal volunteer Phase I study. So we then went back to the drawing board, rewrote our protocol for normal volunteer human subjects, and later conducted that study between 1993 and 1995 at Harbor-UCLA Medical Center.* We studied eighteen individuals in the clinical research unit at Harbor-UCLA Medical Center utilizing pure, government-grade MDMA. Individuals came in on three occasions: on two occasions they received different dosages of MDMA and on one occasion they received an inactive placebo. The order of these differing drug conditions was randomized. Both the subjects and our research team were blinded for the condition at each experimental drug session.

Physiological Effects, Side Effects, and Complications

CG: We measured physiological reactions, including blood pressure and heart rate. We took blood from an indwelling intravenous catheter every thirty minutes to study pharmacokinetics and neuroendocrine secretion, and we utilized a variety of psychological instruments as well. And at the end of the day we found that our subjects tolerated the MDMA experience very well. Two individuals of the eighteen people did have high blood pressure reactions. This is something one has to be wary of. One was an older individual who simply had labile blood pressure [hypertension]. His baseline blood pressure was normal, but under the influence of the MDMA he did have a significant rise.

The other subject was interesting because he was in his third session, so on at least one other occasion he had received MDMA, and on this third occasion his blood pressure shot up, whereas during the previous two occasions his blood pressure had remained normal. When I asked

---

*C. S. Grob, R. E. Poland, L. Chang, and T. Ernst. "Psychobiologic Effects of 3,4-methylenedioxymethamphetamine (MDMA) in Humans: Methodological Considerations and Preliminary Data," *Behavioural Brain Research* 73 (1996): 103–7.

him if there was anything different about this morning than the previous occasions, he said that although there had been something different he didn't want to bother us by telling us. He went on to say he had stayed at a friend's house overnight who lived close by, to get to the hospital early in the morning. His friend had a cat. The subject was allergic to cats and had some trouble breathing in the morning, so his friend gave him some of his asthma medications. So we learned that interactions with particular medications can potentially be somewhat risky, and individuals do need to be apprised of that.

The Power of the Placebo

CG: We also had one individual who appeared to have experienced an adverse psychological reaction. He got very anxious and said that the hospital was not the right place to be on this kind of drug and that he was picking up on all the bad vibes of the hospital. We talked him down and told him that he could drop out of the study. This was his first session; he could drop out of the study but he had to spend the night in the hospital because he had agreed to that for safety reasons. When he left in the morning he decided he was going to withdraw from the study. So we decided to break the blind to see how much MDMA we had given him to cause such an anxious and fearful kind of response, and to our amazement it turned out we had given him a placebo. So never underestimate the power of the placebo response. The guy had simply psyched himself out.

Initial Results Bode Well for Safety

RLM: You talked about the subjects that had a little difficulty. What about the ones who did not have difficulty?

CG: The nineteenth subject, who never got MDMA, just got the placebo and dropped out. The others did remarkably well. They physiologically tolerated the experience well. Psychologically they had very upbeat, positive experiences. The only other problem I ran into was one day the head nurse on the research unit took me aside and complained that her nurses were spending too much time with my subjects and not enough time with their other patients. I thought they were just enjoying talking with our subjects and almost getting a contact high, or perhaps our subjects were so empathetic and interested in the lives of the nurses that perhaps that made it alluring for them to just spend that time.

But our subjects did very well. We published our results. Although our group at that time did not go on to do any therapeutic studies with MDMA—this had been a normal volunteer study—Michael Mithoefer's group in South Carolina did move the MDMA field forward by doing his controlled studies with chronic PTSD patients.

What's Keeping MDMA Underground?

Lack of Government Funding

RLM: It is interesting to note that the medicine MDMA is called "ecstasy" on the street. The public knows that it has had widespread use and not just in this country but around the world. But on the other hand, we don't really hear about widespread sub rosa use of Prozac. You don't hear of thousands of people going to parties and taking Zoloft, for example. MDMA has been referred to as an empathogen, given that it has the capacity for enhancing empathy, and an entheogen—bringing on a kind of religious experience. Was the government not impressed enough with this research to want to facilitate or support more research?

CG: We've had success since the early '90s with obtaining government regulatory approvals. They often take some time, and there's often a lot of back and forth, but at the end of the day we've found the regulatory agencies to be fairly reasonable. The limiting step is funding.

The national health funding agencies are not prioritizing therapeutic research with psychedelics, so the money has to be raised from private sources. We've completed the studies we've had funding for, and now we are looking at our depleted funding accounts and trying to raise additional funding, but it is a painstakingly laborious process.

Suppression of Doctors' Personal Experience

RLM: In a previous interview you were asked, "Have you ever taken MDMA?" I imagine it would be very tempting for many researchers, when they come across something like MDMA that enhances empathy, to want to take it.

I'm not going to ask if you've ever taken it, but instead I'm going to quote your response, because I think it is terrific: "My response to that sort of question is usually along the lines of 'I'm damned if I have and I'm damned if I haven't.'"

This is very accurate: "If I have taken ecstasy then my perspective as a researcher would be discounted due to my own personal-use bias, and if I haven't taken it I would be discounted because I would not truly understand the full range of experience the drug can induce."

I imagine that's an issue for all research, as in all of these various medicines, isn't it?

CG: Yes, I've taken the tack of not responding to those questions but rather just pointing out the dilemma that each answer would lead to.

RLM: Yes, of course. Since I'm not a researcher in the area I can tell you that I was given MDMA in my doctor's office back before it was scheduled, and it had a very helpful effect on me. I had repeated sessions with him. Your quote about how it may induce profound psychological realignments that could take decades to achieve on my therapist's couch without it was absolutely correct; it was a huge benefit. I could immediately see the benefits for people all over the world, undoubtedly. It was so obvious, and so it has been painful to see how little research is going on.

Advice for Personal Experimentation

RLM: You and I differentiate between a material used as a medicine and the exact same material used as a drug. We know that there are people using LSD, MDMA, and psilocybin recreationally, and we also know that people are using the same exact materials as medicines—like it or not, whether the government likes it or not, and whether we are concerned about these folks or not. This is going on, and it's happening on a widespread scale. Many listeners are experimenting in their own lives. What can you say, in terms of caution or encouragement, to the people who are going to do this regardless of what you or the government have to say?

CG: It certainly would be a lot easier to have these compounds thoroughly examined and vetted for treatment modalities if there was no recreational use going on, but that's not the real world we live in. There are a lot of people who are drawn to these compounds for a variety of reasons. They need to understand that they could get into serious difficulty. There are significant adverse medical effects that can occur with MDMA or ecstasy use.

These effects are aggravated by common settings where it's taken. People are exercising vigorously at dances, in crowded or stuffy environments. They forget to replace body fluids, and you can get the malignant hyperthermia catastrophes. On the flip side, individuals who are not exercising but are drinking copious quantities of water, particularly women, may expose themselves to a life-threatening water intoxication syndrome.

I'm a big supporter of the harm-reduction model. You take it as a given that individuals are going to be inquisitive, so you just try to provide them with essential information that will lessen the likelihood that they could harm themselves. You want to help people be more risk avoidant.

•••

My next interview regarding MDMA is with another person I consider a friend, Phil Wolfson, MD. Wolfson is a psychiatrist, researcher, author, political activist, and gardener. His book, *The Ketamine Papers,* was the subject of a recent TV-and-radio interview we did together. I am pleased to present here Phil's insights into his work with MDMA.

Demonstrating MDMA's Safety and Efficacy in Treating End-of-Life Anxiety
Phil Wolfson, MD
December 2, 2014

PHIL WOLFSON, MD, earned his BA at Brandeis University. He went on to medical school at New York University School of Medicine and began practicing psychotherapy and psychiatry in the Bay Area in 1977. He is licensed to practice medicine in California and Washington, DC. Dr. Wolfson has been an assistant clinical professor of psychiatry at the University of California San Francisco and has taught at several graduate schools. He was one of the founding members of the Heffter Research Institute, which is another psychedelic research organization, along with MAPS, the Multidisciplinary Association for Psychedelic Studies. He is the author of *Noe: A Father-Son Song of Love, Life, Illness, and Death* and is editor/contributor of *The Ketamine Papers.*

Dr. Wolfson is the principal investigator of a double-blind, placebo-controlled Phase II study located in Marin, California, which is in the middle of its work concerning the safety and efficacy of MDMA-assisted psychotherapy for anxiety in eighteen subjects diagnosed with a life-threatening illness. The study has received coverage in the *San Francisco Chronicle* and on KQED Radio's *Forum* with Michael Krasny as well as in media around the globe, and it is bringing more mainstream attention to the topic of psychedelic medicines, psychedelic psychotherapy, and legalization.

Called to Help and Be Helped
Early MDMA Treatments for the Chemically Wounded

RLM: Dr. Phil Wolfson was recently granted FDA approval to use MDMA legally in his psychotherapy practice. Tell us about that please, Phil.

Phil Wolfson, MD (PW): I was running an alternative psychiatric unit in Contra Costa County called I Ward, which was based on the notion that people in altered states of consciousness could benefit from work with their actual state of psychosis, using family members and supportive teams, and going through the course of their mental alteration. This would apply to first-break schizophrenia and to some degree bipolar illness. I had a very difficult patient who had been seriously wounded, chemically, by mega dosages of the neuroleptic drugs in use at the time. I was looking for an alternative substance when I was introduced to Sasha Shulgin, the great psychochemist. I visited him, and he suggested the use of MDMA. As it was legal in those days, he and his wife Anne gave me a session with my wife. I began to see its utility as what we came to call an empathogen—a substance that elicited warmth, closeness, and an ability to better handle negative emotions and to find compassion for self and others.

A large number of psychotherapists and psychiatrists, including myself, began to use MDMA in our clinical practices, which was in many respects a revolution in psychotherapy and psychiatry, because you had to sit with people for long periods of time. You could do open work with process, and the sessions could last anywhere from three to five hours, or longer, and you had to stay with people until their process concluded. It was a fantastic opportunity, really, to get to know people and elicit new kinds of consciousness and reactions.

A Family Copes with Tragedy

RLM: What can you tell us from your memory of your first session with MDMA when Shulgin and his wife administered it to you?

PW: I was not a naive subject—I had done my first trip with LSD in 1964 while in medical school. MDMA was quite a bit different. It was not hallucinogenic; it was warm. It was relatively easy to work with, to stay in touch, and in many respects it was what came to be called a love drug. It was an exciting way to be with people—to be deeper in oneself and to handle negativity, judgments, and reactions that might have been obsessional or interfering with relationships. My session was a very close and warm session with people I hardly knew, who were just generous, thoughtful people. It was very helpful to my wife and me.

RLM: Did you and your wife go on to use it together after that?

PW: Well, unfortunately, I had a terrible experience in my life. My eldest son Noah contracted leukemia when he was nearly thirteen. That was the year after that session. I had begun using MDMA in therapy, especially with couples and occasionally with families. During the course of my son's four-year illness, we as a family—the parents, not the children—would have sessions with MDMA in order to bring about a sense of family unity and process, which I actually wrote about in my book about my son's life and illness. So it was very valuable episodic support to our lives and our ability to cope with a terrible illness.

RLM: Please remind us of the name of the book that you wrote about yourself and your son?

PW: It's called *Noe: A Father-Son Song of Love, Life, Illness, and Death.*

DEA Shuts the Lid on MDMA Research
How MDMA Got a Bad Reputation

RLM: You were a licensed psychiatrist using MDMA legally in your practice in California, and then George Ricaurte publishes an article in the very prestigious journal, *Science,* in which he says that MDMA causes neurotoxicity in primates after a common recreational dose regimen. What happened after that?

PW: My memory is a little different, Richard. We were working with larger numbers of people, and MDMA was spreading in a relatively small way when the DEA got into the act in 1984 and insisted on scheduling the drug. The DEA appointed an administrative law judge to have a hearing. We had national press, and a lot of us got up and talked about the merits of MDMA. In fact, the judge found in favor of scheduling MDMA in a still-accessible schedule—Schedule II—within the Federal Regulatory statute. The DEA overruled that—their own judge—and made MDMA illegal in 1985. Subsequently, there was a vast explosion of use. As usual, illegalization had the impact of increasing interest in it.

Ricaurte came later. He was doing so-called science, and he came to the periphery of the group and then toward MAPS, which had formed to scientifically develop an argument against the DEA's scheduling by showing the utility, scientifically and clinically, of MDMA. In that process, Ricaurte, as with others before him, had been making a reputation by basically doing pseudoscience and cultivating a negativity that would give him a reputation through the Drug Enforcement Agency and give him authority, money, and position.

As it evolved, he came toward us looking for experienced subjects that he could test in a variety of ways. As he was writing negative stories about the serotonergic problems with MDMA, he gained stature among the naysayers and war-on-drugs folks, and then he published in *Science* after getting that stature.

It turned out that he and his group were so-called "mistakenly" using methamphetamine in their studies—at least two of them, but I believe there were others—and he was forced to retract the data that implicated MDMA. Unfortunately, dirty work persists and dirty minds have an effect, and the negativity toward MDMA continued.

What was not talked about—it is always interesting to me—is that methamphetamine is a dopaminergic substance. It works on the dopamine neurotransmitter primarily, whereas MDMA worked on the serotonin neurotransmitter primarily, and secondarily norepinephrine and perhaps dopamine. So here he was writing about the serotonergic effects of methamphetamine, which doesn't have any; so the whole thing was a terrible abuse of science and caused quite a stir.

RLM: It caused a tremendous stir and it left the public with the impression that MDMA is far more hazardous than it turned out to be. Both Congress and the former director of the National Institute of Drug Abuse, Alan Leshner, came out strongly about how dangerous MDMA was even after Ricaurte was forced to retract his entire mistaken article. British scientists went on record expressing their concerns, Phil. I have a quote: "It's an outrageous scandal," Leslie Iverson said, "It's another example of a certain breed of scientist who appears to do research on illegal drugs mainly to show what the governments want them to show. They extract large amounts of grant money from the government to do this sort of biased work."* That's quite an indictment.

PW: You beat me to the quote. I had that in front of me. When I was in med school in the heyday of LSD, there was a guy at New York University making a reputation by finding chromosomal breaks caused by LSD, which was bogus work. He did very well by giving the negative camp ammunition and then eventually that was retracted. There were no chromosomal breaks. But the impression

---

*Phillip S. Smith, "Newsbrief: Ecstasy Scandal Grows as Second Study Retracted," *Drug War Chronicle* 303 (September 19, 2013).

still lingers—unfortunately. So there is a long history of toady syco-
phants working to make money and a reputation within science. You
always have to look at science with a grain of salt and look at who is
sponsoring whom, and who is going where.

RLM: It's intimidating.

PW: And fascinating.

RLM: And fascinating at the same time. One of the things I didn't tell
the listeners about you is that you're also a Buddhist practitioner. So
these words of wisdom that come out when I say it's intimidating,
and you say it's fascinating, are also delightfully and beautifully from
your Buddhist background, which I very much appreciate.

PW: You are very sweet to me, thank you.

RLM: Well you've always been very sweet to me as well, Phil.

The Bay Area MDMA Study with End-of-Life Anxiety

RLM: I want to move on to a discussion of the historic study that
you're going to be doing, please tell us about it.

PW: Sure, it's an exciting study. We—MAPS—were given a grant by
a man, who unfortunately died, to explore the effects of MDMA-
assisted psychotherapy on anxiety in people with life-threatening
illnesses who are at risk for relapse or recurrence, or death itself.
We've designed the study to maximize the possibility of observing
the effects of MDMA. We have FDA approval that allows us to do
a Phase II study.

There are three phases on the path from science to the prescription.
This is an orphan drug—it has no patent, because it was first patented
in 1914 and that expired many decades ago. Phase I is for assessing
toxicity of a substance. Phase II is to assess both safety and efficacy in

small numbers. Phase III entails a much wider study, which sets the stage for prescriptions by MDs worldwide.

We're in Phase II with MAPS, moving toward Phase III, particularly with studies directed toward post-traumatic stress disorder. Our study in the Bay Area is the first one with MDMA here, and it is attempting to look at anxiety in people who have had a terrible illness and are fearing recurrence, relapse, or death itself, but have a life expectancy ahead of them. We hope that anxiety will be reduced by MDMA-assisted psychotherapy. So it's a very complex approach to working with MDMA in a thoughtful and integrated psychotherapy practice.

This study is probably going to take one and a half to two years because it's complex and involves a randomization—sorting people into groups of subjects who will receive placebos and then go on to MDMA sessions as well as subjects that receive the MDMA from the start. We've designed it so that it includes people who are not terminally ill—who have a life-threatening illness but are not acutely ill. The study, which will take at least four months for each person, can go on without being severely impacted by people's declines or illnesses that may inevitably occur during the study, unfortunately; so the study has a large therapy component. We go through a screening process to accept people, and then we do a series of preliminary sessions followed by overnight sessions. Participants will be at my home for twenty-four hours, where they have a very comfortable and intense experience.

We are working with two institutional review boards. We finished with one and almost with another, and we're waiting for the DEA to come inspect the premises. I've had to put a safe in my house, and we've wired the place because the DEA requires stringent security mechanisms to protect the MDMA that is shipped to us in bulk. We have a formulating pharmacist who makes placebos and identical capsules containing MDMA, which are tracked by computer. I am blinded to their contents—only the computer knows and randomizes.

The computer and MDMA stay in the safe, and the DEA is very concerned about security for that.

RLM: What do you mean when you say you've wired the house?

PW: We have to put an alarm system in, as well as for the room in which the safe is located.

Nonclinical "Anecdata"

RLM: Let me take you back to the time when MDMA was legal, and you were allowed to use it and you did use it as a psychiatrist in your practice. You also must have known other therapists who were using it in their practice. What was the usefulness or the dangers of this medicine back then, prior to its becoming illegal?

PW: It was in small-scale use. By that I mean tens of thousands of doses. Now one estimate has twenty-nine million users in one year, 2012. But it became renowned as a therapy drug. Quite a large number of people using it were practitioners, and we formed some informal organizations to collaborate and exchange data. It was quite persuasive in its use for couples—helping relationships integrate—and people becoming more expressive. We had a lot of people get married on MDMA. We used to warn people not to get married on MDMA: "You're in the glow! Take a little time see if the glow persists after use." But people didn't always listen, and I know of a few marriages that have survived over these decades after an MDMA set of sessions. We used it for individuals with depression, where it had wonderful effects—not 100 percent, but people often got better with a series of MDMA sessions in a psychotherapeutic context. Anxiety often improved. It was a short period, really, from 1982 to 1985—after which it became illegal and research could no longer continue with our informal network—but there were lots of publications, and many people were influenced by their experience with MDMA in a positive way.

Looking Critically at Risks

Side Effects, Dangerous Mixtures, and Overdose

RLM: People are hearing this, Phil, and they're learning about thousands of people who took MDMA in their therapist's office between 1979 and 1985. They are also learning that twenty-nine million people have used it recreationally in one year—in one year, twenty-nine million people! So people may be saying to themselves that this sounds like something they'd like to try. We have the responsibility to tell them what might happen that's not very pleasant. Were there problems or negative side effects from using MDMA?

PW: It's really important for people to be informed users. In general, the substance is quite safe. Mixing it with other substances has been the biggest cause of problems. In fact, most of the deaths attributed to MDMA are the result of a mix of substances ranging from alcohol to methamphetamine and other unspecified contaminants used to reduce cost to the dealer.

The number of actual deaths related to *pure* MDMA itself used in good settings can be characterized as truly rare, but still present, so there is some risk as with any substance. You want to be in a good set and setting. You want to be with people who are responsible and who can help you in case of emergency. An emergency almost never happens with a good set and setting. In our set of studies of over nine hundred people, there have been no significant medical problems. That's within the MAPS set of studies. So the things to watch out for are getting too hot—MDMA and MDA substances that are related to amphetamines or methamphetamines can cause a heat problem, so you want to cool off—and mixing substances can be problematic.

There are always minor side effects to begin with, such as jaw clenching and headache. Some people speak of a kind of emptiness or grayness, which can persist for a couple days, or even a mid-week low. I have never seen that in my extensive use, but it is reported. There is dehydration if you don't drink enough—and that was a source of problems that came up during the illegal period at raves where people were in high-heat environments and didn't drink properly. There were several deaths. And there was also the rare problem of overhydration. During the legal period, we saw one strange reaction I could not explain, in which a person on a known batch of MDMA ended up in the ICU with a neurological illness. She fully recovered, but there was no explanation for that. So, like with all drugs, there is a certain level of risk of idiosyncratic reactions.

There is also a question of whether there's such a thing as MDMA overdose. There has been an unverified report of a death in England of a young girl—a tragic death—of a fifteen-year-old who weighed one hundred pounds and took 500 milligrams, which is four times the usual dosage. There are issues of purity that come up as well. This girl apparently was in a group that got a powerful, new, and purer MDMA substance. The dilution of MDMA has been extreme in many cases, so people were getting pills and tablets that might have had 25 to 30 percent MDMA, or even less, with another dilutant. One issue for consumers is to know what you're getting.

RLM: Can you recommend a place where people can send something they buy and get an honest analysis so they know what it is they're taking, since they're not allowed to buy it legally at the drugstore?

PW: Well, the most beneficial one is called DanceSafe, which does analyses. I'm not sure of the current status of other testing agencies. I can't recommend one, but DanceSafe was established to make sure that there was safety among users at raves and parties. It was done entirely for the benefit of people, without money being an issue. It's a worthy thing to look up, and you can purchase kits to assess the presence of many different substances. So you can examine for purity.

RLM: And there's also a website called Erowid.org that has intellectual content to read.

PW: If you really want to know about what you're doing and what you're taking, if you want to read user reports and get a sense of what's going on currently in the world of psychoactive drugs, go to Erowid. They are great people and they're doing a great service.

Controlling the Set and Setting

RLM: Earlier in the program you said that as long as the set and setting were appropriate, this is a very safe medicine. Please elaborate on the words *set* and *setting* and what they mean to our listeners?

PW: Well, setting is the obvious one. Be in a comfortable, safe place with support when you do substances. People I know who have gotten into trouble—kids and others—have been out in the world in places where heightened vigilance is necessary, because they're doing something that makes them more wary and puts them in the view of police, and so forth.

The set idea is what you bring to it—your own mental status, your own view of things, where you are with yourself. It's a very good practice before using a psychedelic substance to spend the day getting clear and clean, to prepare yourself to make it a sacred experience—one that recognizes the power of what you're going to do and doesn't just take it for granted. When you take that time—when you prepare yourself, when you meditate, when you do some exercise or yoga before, when you really set the stage, light candles, and create an environment that is conducive to your use—your exploration is going to go deeper and your safety will be much better.

RLM: So you're talking about the difference between creating an ambience, a setting, and preparing a mental set, so that you're taking the substance as *medicine* rather than "doing drugs."

PW: Yeah, I'd say that's a good idea. A vast number of people have gotten away with doing drugs and have gotten myriad benefits from it, but if you want to improve your odds, do it the way we just discussed.

RLM: Now given people are hearing this and they're going to perhaps experiment, some people suggest that when you do this in the privacy of your own home you should not do certain things such as answer the telephone or turn on the television set or go to the front door and start talking to people who happen to be in the neighborhood. How do you feel about those things and what other kinds of privacy or safeguards might you recommend?

PW: Well, it's good to turn the cell phone off. It's good to not get distracted by things that are silly. I think having great music is always a benefit. It's deepening to have instruments, where you might play drums or bells. I love bells. I think the sound of bells is penetrating and overcomes obsession and other preoccupations. Do not operate motor vehicles or heavy-duty machinery.

Take the time to make the space solid and take the time afterward to integrate. A lot of us talk about integrative work for sessions after an experience. Take the time to look at your experience, remember it as best as possible, and take some notes for your own benefit, because memory does fade and it's sometimes hard to recover the memory of the experience.

MDMA's Relation to Amphetamines

RLM: We're going to take a caller here, Phil.

Caller: Hi, thanks for your program.

RLM: You're welcome.

Caller: I have heard of MDA [methylenedioxyamphetamine], and I would rather not have the side effects of methamphetamine, so I'm wondering if there is a pure substance that you are working with that works without the methamphetamine. Thank you.

PW: I can point out to you something that is easily confused—look at the chemical pictures of both methamphetamine and MDA if you can. MDA is amphetamine. The difference is that the MDA molecule has the amphetamine structure, whereas methamphetamine has the CH_3 group on another part of it. Neither the substance MDA nor MDMA resembles amphetamine or methamphetamine in side effects—only partially at best.

Amphetamine and methamphetamine both have pretty similar side effects. Hyperthermia, or too high of a temperature, and jaw clench are problems with both substances. So anything related structurally to amphetamine, such as methamphetamine, will have some of those side effects. That said, they are very different molecules and they have very different effects. Mescaline is in the same framework—there are myriad psychoactive substances that are related to those. If you look further you'll see that many of the spices on your shelf also have very similar structures; so the structural analysis of molecules and their effects on the mind is very intricate and not straightforward.

Emergency Room Visits from MDMA

RLM: When we had the last cocaine epidemic, which goes in cycles of about twenty years or so, there were reports from all over the United States of emergency room admissions of people taking overdoses of cocaine. You tell us that approximately twenty-nine million people used MDMA last year. Are we getting admission reports from emergency rooms as a result of this MDMA use, or not?

PW: There are some great statistics. There is a very interesting online group called the DEA.org [Davis Education Association], if you really want to look at statistics for the last period of reporting. I'm looking at it as we speak, and there were 5,542 visits to emergency rooms across the United States; that's in 2001. Apparently we don't have more recent data.

If you take a look at the SSRI Paxil [paroxetine], where I would imagine there is much less use, that's 8,932 use visits. For amphetamine, it lists 8,000. For nonsteroidals—ibuprofen, Naprosyn, Aleve, Advil, and so forth—the number is 22,000. For all antidepressants it's 61,000. Those MDMA numbers apply also to other drugs that are being used along with MDMA, so it's not a pure statistic. People go in for anxiety reactions and physical reactions of various sorts.

RLM: The 61,000 emergency room admissions for people on antidepressants sort of ties in with a guest we had a few weeks ago, Robert Whitaker, and his book *Anatomy of an Epidemic,* in which he talks about his research indicating that antidepressants are causing mental illness [see chapter 5].

Underworld Production of Synthetic Drugs

RLM: Let's take this call here. Welcome to *Mind, Body, Health & Politics.* You're on the air.

Caller: Where is ecstasy being produced? Is it coming from laboratories and then being black marketed, or are there people cooking it up in a back room?

PW: The production of ecstasy is across the world including the United States. Some is apparently coming in from China. There are stories of North Korea making drugs of various sorts, which I think could be true, and India is also a source. There are chemists within countries such as the United Kingdom—and all across our country and the globe.

RLM: So, if I understand you correctly, when it comes to illegal substances, until we analyze what we have before us we cannot know what we have; caveat emptor. Is MDMA difficult to make?

PW: MDMA is difficult. You need precursors, and precursors are tightly controlled. I'm not an authority on how easy or difficult it is to make.

RLM: And what about the use of MDMA concurrently with other psychedelic substances? We have a few minutes left. Please tell us a little about that.

PW: Sure. It's quite common for people to do an admixture; that is, to take more than one substance together to try to affect the nature of their individual effects. So it's common use, for instance, to take MDMA with LSD. MDMA is used with many other substances to make them a bit smoother.

Is MDMA a Sex Drug?

RLM: I have a question here that was handed to me. Is MDMA a sex drug?

PW: It depends who you talk to. MDMA is an extremely sensual substance. The general idea out there is that it doesn't lead to sex. I would argue with that—it may well lead to sex, and it may well lead to lovely sex. It's pretty difficult for people to have an orgasm on MDMA, but I'm sure some people have achieved that. When we did the first study of MDMA, which was in 1994 in a wonderful home in Stinson Beach, I was one of the people designing the study and not taking the substance. It was very difficult to proceed with the neurological and mental statuses I was doing with the twenty or so subjects there, because they were just hugging and kissing and touching, so it was very hard to get attention.

RLM: Since it does affect blood pressure, what about the use of MDMA with Viagra and Cialis, which also lower blood pressure? Is that going to create a problem?

PW: I can't answer that question. I don't have enough information on that.[*]

---

[*]For more information on interactions between MDMA and erectile-dysfunction drugs see "Sildenafil (Viagra) & MDMA (Ecstasy)," Erowid.org, v1.1, March 29, 2012, https://erowid.org/chemicals/mdma/mdma_health7.shtml (accessed April 30, 2017).

RLM: But as far as MDMA's raising blood pressure, that has not been a concern in leading to emergency room visits?

PW: Not that I'm aware of. There is a reliable and definite increase in blood pressure, pulse rate, and temperature with MDMA use, but generally without severity and with quick return to baseline.

Bottom Line: Get Educated

RLM: We're reaching the end of our interview. Is there any last-minute thing you might want to mention to our listeners about MDMA?

PW: For more information, our website at MAPS—the Multidisciplinary Association for Psychedelic Studies—is terrific. Erowid.org is also a great source of information. Be thoughtful about your use and remember, *it is still illegal*. We just passed Proposition 47 in California that really reduces penalties for possession. Look at the terms of Proposition 47 and understand that it's a major change in our drug prohibition policy, locally.

I have been delighted to be with you, Richard. Thank you so much.

•••

A Husband and Wife Team for MDMA Research

I met psychiatrist and researcher Michael Mithoefer, MD, ten years ago when he and I joined June Ruse, PhD, José Carlos Bouso Saiz, PhD, and Peter Cohen on a scientific trip to Israel organized by Rick Doblin, PhD, the founder of MAPS. The purpose of the trip was to ask the Israelis to allow research into the use of MDMA for PTSD, which they recently have allowed.

Here in the United States, Michael and his wife, Annie, were involved with some of the very first research on MDMA, which was sponsored by MAPS. The Mithoefers are currently conducting MDMA research at their facility in Charleston, South Carolina, and Michael is also the medical monitor for MAPS-sponsored clinical trials in Europe, the Middle East, Canada, and Colorado. I am pleased to include the following interview with them.

MDMA for Post-traumatic Stress Disorder

Michael Mithoefer, MD, and Annie Mithoefer, BSN

October 4, 2011

MICHAEL MITHOEFER, MD, spent a decade of his early career as a board-certified emergency medical physician. He is certified in internal medicine, and in 1991 he became certified in psychiatry. He and Annie Mithoefer, BSN, have a private practice of psychiatry in clinical research in Mount Pleasant, South Carolina. On November 2, 2001, Michael and Annie obtained FDA approval to run a clinical trial in the United States giving MDMA in combination with psychotherapy to treat chronic, treatment-resistant post-traumatic stress disorder. The first experimental session of this Phase II clinical trial happened in April of 2004. This is a historic, groundbreaking study.

Overcoming Research Suppression
Politics Triumphs over Science

RLM: Annie, how did you and Michael get interested in MDMA?

Annie Mithoefer, BSN (AM): We experienced MDMA with a therapist when it was legal and did some couples work and found it to be incredibly useful. We did holotropic breathwork training together and learned how you can use techniques to help people process things like trauma, which started our curiosity about it.

RLM: You had a personal experience while MDMA was still a legal medicine in this country, and you were so impressed with the value that you got from the medicine that it sparked your scientific interest; is that what you're saying?

AM: It did spark our scientific interest. We have also worked with many people who have had trauma or difficult times in their lives, and because of this we were constantly looking for something new to help people since many people are not helped by traditional therapies.

RLM: When did MDMA move from being a legal medicine to being categorized by our government as an illegal medicine; or, when did it get turned into what's called a "drug" instead of a medicine?

Michael Mithoefer, MD (MM): That was in 1985 when the DEA put MDMA in Schedule I. Actually, this was contrary to the recommendations of the administrative law judge who ran the hearings about MDMA, who recommended that it should be a prescription medicine. The DEA at that time overruled that recommendation and put it in Schedule I. It was first patented in 1914 by Merck, but they never used it for anything. It was used as an adjunct to therapy when it was legal in the 1970s, but in 1985 all legal use came to an end.

RLM: Annie and Michael, you both first experienced this medicine when you were patients in a therapist office while the medicine was legal, and you had a positive experience. I'll share with you that in 1983 I was administered MDMA in my therapist's office. I had it over a series of sessions and found that it was profoundly helpful in my own personal growth and development. In your opinions, why did the government take this position on something that you, Annie, a psychiatric nurse, and you, Michael, a psychiatrist, and I, a doctor of clinical psychology, have all used to our benefit?

MM: I don't know the answer to that, but it must have been political rather than scientific. There was concern that use had spread to selling it in bars and for recreational use. And the government was, I'm sure, reacting in part to that. It was striking in the hearings—there were very reputable medical professionals testifying on its potential safe use in therapeutic hands, with Dr. Charlie Grob, a psychiatrist from UCLA, being one of those. There was no question in the hearings that there were reasons it should be further researched, so I can only conclude that it was a political decision.

There's a lot of fear, and also there is the drug-war mentality—some people are afraid of sending the wrong message. If you allow for the fact that some things may be dangerous when used unwisely but also may be very useful, healing, and even lifesaving when used by health professionals, that's a more complicated message than just "all drugs are bad."

RLM: Would you be willing to go a little further in your speculation as to what you mean by a political decision? Here we have something that, as far as I know, there have been very few if any incidences of emergency room admissions around the country, particularly when MDMA is used as a medicine. Was the risk theological? Where do you think they were coming from in the suppression, particularly of the research? It's really a head-scratcher.

MM: It is a head-scratcher. There was a lot of promising psychedelic research going on in the '50s and '60s and early '70s, but then President Richard Nixon took a strong position in favor of the drug war, and the government turned away from funding or even allowing most research with these compounds. It was very irrational from a medical point of view.

Suppressed but Not Banned

RLM: How is it that some of these medicines are not only researched but also are sold to the public and then some of them such as MDMA are selected out—not only are they made illegal for consumption, but research at the university level is also made illegal?

MM: It's fascinating. I scratch my head too, although the research hasn't actually been made illegal. It was more of a de facto thing. In fact, people couldn't get studies approved or funded for many years.

RLM: Fifty years later, and I stand corrected—you're right—it's not that the research was made illegal. It's just that the research was suppressed.

MM: Right. It just isn't tenable to say there is a group of potential medicines that might be very helpful for these people who aren't responding to the existing therapies, but we're not allowed to even look there. That's just not a tenable position for a physician or a psychologist or a nurse to be in. We need to look for anything that sounds like it might be promising without prejudice—according to scientific data, not political decisions.

RLM: Yes. In fact, not only are we not able to offer people these medicines, we're not even able to tell people where in the world they might go to obtain them. In other areas of medicine, you can send people to another country if they want to be on the cutting edge. But in this particular case, we can't even do that because the United States government suppresses the research in other areas of the world.

I had the good fortune to be with Michael Mithoefer some years ago as part of a small expedition of scientists that went to Israel to talk with their scientists about the use of MDMA with people suffering from PTSD—post-traumatic stress disorder—particularly during the Intifada, when there were body parts flying around and people were severely traumatized. I'm sure you'll bear this out, Michael, that we were told that although the Israelis were interested in doing this research, they really couldn't until the United States gave them the go-ahead, because they could lose funding. Correct?

MM: I recall that. I don't recall if they said the exact reason. But they did make it clear that they wouldn't consider it until we had full approval for our research here.

RLM: Extraordinary suppression, as you said.

Hopeful Horizons

MM: The good news is that we have been allowed to do research now, and it is picking up. So as you say, we submitted our FDA application in the fall of 2001, in October, and then we got permission from the FDA within thirty days. It then took another two and a half years to get permission from an institutional review board and the DEA. But we were then able to do the first clinical study of MDMA to have been completed.

There were some other studies before us called Phase I trials. Charlie Grob at UCLA did the first of those. Then there were two others in the United States and some in Europe. There was some data about giving it to humans but not for treatment, and there had been one study started in Spain that was shut down. So ours was the first that was actually able to study MDMA as a treatment and be completed. We started in 2004, and one of the important things about this model is that we're not just doing a drug study, but rather we're studying MDMA-assisted psychotherapy. So people don't get MDMA to take home. They get MDMA two or three times, a month apart, in an all-day session with me and Annie as cotherapists.

RLM: This is a medicine that they took in the office with Dr. Mithoefer and his wife Annie, a psychiatric nurse—that's important. Also, the medicine was taken in conjunction with verbal psychotherapy. This was not a medicine that you swallowed and then immediately looked at the results.

MM: There was also careful screening to make sure people didn't have some underlying health problem that might make MDMA dangerous, because it does increase blood pressure and pulse. We monitored those things very carefully. So it is a very controlled setting.

Is MDMA Rightly Considered a Psychedelic?

Entheogens, Entactogens, and Empathogens

RLM: Michael, what do you mean when you refer to a medicine as psychedelic?

MM: Well, I wish we had a better term that was agreed upon. Psychedelic means mind-manifesting, and for many people it implies hallucinations and maybe very strong transpersonal or spiritual kinds of experiences—the kind that you associate with LSD or psilocybin.

RLM: But not with MDMA?

MM: MDMA is different. Some people have suggested other terms like entactogen, something that helps you touch within, or empathogen, something that increases empathy.

RLM: Or entheogen. It gives sort of a mystical, almost religious experience. But no one has pointed a finger at this particular medicine MDMA and accused it of being a hallucination- or schizophrenic-mimetic or anything like that.

MM: No—the terms are often used loosely but you're right. It's quite different and many of these compounds have great potential and need to be studied, and some are being studied; but I think MDMA in some ways is easier to work with clinically, in that it doesn't cause as much of a shift in consciousness as these others do.

Pharmacodynamics of MDMA

MM: MDMA is a molecule that looks something like methamphetamine and something like mescaline. It's a medicine that's taken by mouth in capsule form, as a powder, and it has a wide range of effects on the brain and body.

It largely boils down to a lot of monoamine release—release of things like serotonin, dopamine, and norepinephrine, as well as a number of hormones like prolactin and oxytocin. Basically, it amounts to giving people an experience that's not quite psychedelic in the sense that people often mean—in that it doesn't cause hallucinations. But it does cause a real shift in consciousness that often involves greater insight, greater empathy for self or others, and greater connection with emotions in an interesting way.

It seems to allow people to access difficult emotions that they've been cut off from, but with the sense that they won't be overwhelmed by fear. It also allows access to positive emotions people have been cut off from. So it seems to modulate the emotions in a way that creates a state that's potentially very useful.

RLM: Does MDMA work on the neurotransmitters in the brain in a similar way that legal medicines such as the SSRIs, like Prozac [fluoxetine], Luvox [fluvoxamine], Zoloft [sertraline], Paxil, and so on, do?

MM: Part of the effect is similar in that it does cause changes in the serotonin system in blocking serotonin reuptake, but then there are all these other effects, and no one really understands how they all combine to cause this shift in consciousness.

RLM: We're on the cutting edge, in other words. We're learning about the way these different medicines interact with the neurotransmitters with brain function?

MM: Absolutely. There's a lot to be learned.

Overcoming Treatment-Resistant PTSD

Comparing Against Baseline Ineffective Treatment

RLM: Okay, let's come back to your study.

MM: The first study was with twenty participants, all of whom had treatment-resistant PTSD. And they had to have had prior treatment with both medications—Zoloft and Paxil—that are the two existing treatments approved by the FDA for PTSD or other medicines in the same class. They had to have had at least a course of treatment with these, but most of them had already had many different medicines. And they had to have had at least six months of psychotherapy, and most had more than that. They had to still show significant PTSD symptoms.

RLM: This is how you define "treatment resistant"—meaning they had these various other forms of treatment, and they did not get a significant enough improvement to feel healed or to have gained a sense of well-being.

MM: Right. Part of the study consisted of an independent rater who determined the participants' levels of PTSD before and then later. If people qualified for the study we would do several introductory sessions to get to know them and to prepare them for the experience. Then, after their all-day experience with us, they would spend the night in the clinic with a nurse on duty. We would meet with them the next morning for a ninety-minute session, and we would talk to them every day on the phone for a week. We would meet with them approximately every week for a month in between the sessions to help them integrate the experience.

This study was a double-blind, meaning people got either MDMA on two occasions, one month apart, or placebo on those two occasions, with all the same therapy—the same all-day sessions and the same follow-up treatment. So neither the participants, nor Annie and I, nor the testing psychologist knew who was going to get what. When we broke the blind after we measured their symptoms two months later, if it turned out they'd gotten a placebo then they could go through the whole thing again with MDMA in an open-label fashion so everybody knew what they were getting. That way we could compare how they did with the placebo and how they did when MDMA was added.

Active vs. Inactive Placebo

RLM: Did you use neutral placebos or active placebos?

MM: We used an inactive placebo on this first study.

RLM: The reason I brought that up is because Robert Whitaker, *Anatomy of an Epidemic,* and Irving Kirsch, *The Emperor's New Drugs,* have made some breakthrough studies comparing placebos to the SSRIs, and one of the things they found is that there was a significant difference in results when they used either active or inactive placebos—when they used active placebos, the placebos did much better than the SSRIs.

MM: Yeah. Now, in our current study with veterans, we are using an active placebo.

RLM: Michael is talking about a double-blind study. That means the person who is administering either the medicine or the placebo does not know what each subject is receiving. This procedure is used because it has been found that the mind is so powerful that when the person who hands the medicine to the patient in the study knows what they're giving, it actually has an effect. The person who's doing the administration must be blinded, that is, have no idea who's getting the placebo and who's getting the medicine.

Whitaker, Kirsch, and others have discovered that when you give a neutral, inactive placebo—a sugar pill that has no effect—to some, and you give a medicine to the other people, the people who get the placebo know they're getting the placebo because they feel that nothing happens. And the people who get the medicine know they're getting a medicine, because within a certain number of minutes they can feel something happening.

Therefore, the study itself is affected by our minds knowing, "Oh, I'm one of those who is getting the placebo," or, "Oh, I'm one of those getting the medicine." So these scientists have created placebos that give you a feeling of some kind—not a feeling that alters your mind in any way. It's just a feeling. These placebos that create a feeling are called active placebos. Thus the subjects themselves can't tell which of them are on the medicine and which are on the placebo, because everybody's getting some subjective change in their feeling state.

MM: That's an important point, and we're addressing that in this current study. We felt for other reasons it was important to use an inactive placebo for the first study so that we could really document the differences in side effects. So people would have their two or three sessions, and then, two months after their last MDMA or placebo-assisted session, they would have the PTSD-symptom measures done again by the psychologist. Then we would break the blind, and if it turned out they had received the placebo, then they could go through the same thing again but with active MDMA, and we'd measure the results two months after that. We compared the placebo group and the MDMA group first, and then we also compared the original placebo group's placebo results to that same group's MDMA results.

Encouraging Results

RLM: And what did you discover?

MM: We had very strong, encouraging results. We had a significant effect with placebo in these all-day sessions with all the follow-up therapy. Two of the eight people who received randomized placebo had a very strong placebo response from just that. One of those was fairly short lived, but we did have two strong placebo responders, and the rest did not change or didn't change much. Some got slightly worse and some got a little better with the placebo, but overall the placebo did make a difference. The MDMA group had a much stronger response. In the MDMA group, 83 percent had a very strong clinical response compared to the 25 percent in the placebo group. Then when the placebo group crossed over and had MDMA, everyone had a significant response, including the ones that had no response to the placebo.

The Therapeutic Process: The Struggle Before the Healing

RLM: Annie, did any of the people have a negative response?

AM: No. Sometimes things can look worse at first, as you're digging deeper into the trauma and you're re-experiencing what it feels like to have emotions again. But that would be the only thing that may have been negative in that way. That is why we have so many integration sessions and phone calls every day for a week, because you're helping people move through the trauma.

RLM: And in terms of your measurements, did any of the people score as if they were worse off after the medicine than they were before?

AM: No, not in the PTSD measurements. What I'm talking about is an increase in anxiety a few days after they are back home, when they are thinking about what they talked about and thinking that maybe they shouldn't have talked about it.

RLM: Yes—the middle road before they get to the place of being healed.

MM: Yes, and that's why the integration sessions, we think, are so important to help people move through that period.

PTSD: The Nature of the Beast

RLM: I just realized we've been using the acronym PTSD—post-traumatic stress disorder—but I think it would be a good idea if you two would talk a little bit about PTSD and what it is.

MM: PTSD is a syndrome that sometimes occurs following severe trauma. In this first study it was mostly childhood sexual abuse or rape as an adult, and in the current study it is veterans with either war trauma or military sexual assault. Some people have symptoms but improve without treatment, while a certain percentage of people end up with this thing called PTSD.

The three symptoms clusters are: one, re-experiencing—they either have intrusive memories, flashbacks, or nightmares about the trauma; two, a physiological response to certain cues with hyperarousal, anxiety, startle response, sleep disturbance, and things like that; and three, avoidance—they avoid places and people that remind them of the trauma, or it can also be an inner avoidance, a kind of emotional numbing, i.e., they stay away from emotions because they're upsetting. It's always a combination of those things that we define as PTSD, and it can be very debilitating. Some of the people in the study hardly got out of their house and really could not function well at all. It interfered with their relationships and their physical health. There is very good evidence showing how much more medical morbidity there is in people with PTSD compared to those without it. Many are immobilized by fear and do not want to be with people.

Striking Results: Emotions as a Map to Healing

RLM: You've now gone through the first study. What can you share with the listeners regarding the efficacy of this medicine?

MM: Well, as scientists, we need to keep in mind that this was a small study, even though we found very statistically significant results. We don't want to get ahead of ourselves. We need to see if this can be replicated in larger studies. Having said that, the effect we've seen so far was very striking and encouraging. People have told us it changed their relationship with their emotions.

RLM: Say more about that, Annie. Please speak to that topic.

AM: They are usually so afraid to revisit the traumatic event or the emotions that are around it that they completely shut everything out.

What sometimes happens in the MDMA session is that they have an experience of some emotion coming, and with your help, they can sit with it and they can realize they are able to deal with these feelings. I think another thing that happens for people is a template of feeling really good and relaxed, like they have never felt in their whole life. Just having that template and helping people anchor that within themselves, then they can go back to it—like a map for this good feeling.

RLM: It makes sense. If I understand, you're saying that the traumatic experience was so powerful in one area of emotion that, as a protective device against the pain of that experience, all emotions were blanketed out. Is that what you're saying?

AM: Exactly.

RLM: So they're walking around in a state of constantly or automatically having to suppress one of the most vital aspects of the human condition, which is our emotional state.

AM: Yes.

RLM: And the medicine, with your guidance and help in therapy, allows subjective feeling and/or expression of an emotion, which then opens the door for an experience. Is that correct?

MM: Yes.

Climbing Down Ladders to Dark Feelings
Facing Anxiety without Being Taken Over

RLM: We've got another caller here. Welcome to *Mind, Body, Health & Politics*. You're on the air.

Caller: Good morning. What is it actually like to experience this chemical as it begins to affect you?

AM: For some people, when the drug comes on it can make them more anxious. There's a little bit of time when we talk people through that, and we have them use their breath. This is usually when the medicine is coming on initially. Then the positive effects of the medicine gradually set in, and they aren't as fearful—they aren't thinking about that anxiety. In the beginning, the effects focus patients and bring them into the present moment in a way that they've never experienced before. It often brings up things from their childhood and positive things in their lives, such as surviving the trauma or having a family that loves them. And then it will open up—it's different for each person—and sometimes they will have very strong stories and pictures that go with their experience, where they have an animal that comes to them and talks them through it or there might be images such as looking in jars that hold the trauma.

MM: Some people would see images during their MDMA sessions. One was as if the trauma were down in this dark place, and the MDMA gave them ladders so they could descend into the feelings. It was painful, but they could go there; it allowed them to process and integrate these emotions without being taken over by them.

AM: And what Michael means by "being taken over by it" is the tendency for people to react with fear, anger, or rage to these memories.

MM: Sometimes there's a comfortable feeling in the body, so it can be quite affirming. People with PTSD often haven't felt comfortable in their body since the trauma. One person told us that after having been abused as a child, he had never felt happiness—he only deduced what it must be from watching other people's behavior. He felt happiness for the first time with MDMA. He realized it was actually a possibility for him. So there's that very comfortable, positive part of it.

But often it was very difficult, and a lot of people told us they didn't know why it was called ecstasy because a lot of time was spent revisiting trauma and having painful feelings that were still very difficult. In a nutshell, what's effective about MDMA is that people can revisit the trauma and not be emotionally cut off from it. They still have the pain. They still have to move through the feelings, but it gives them a sense that they can work through it. So the experience seems to be a combination of those affirming, positive, and comfortable experiences with the more painful ones that they are able to process in a more helpful way.

RLM: I'll go back some twenty-eight years to the experience in my therapist's office. I recall that the experience I had, as this medicine saturated my system, was a feeling of connecting with what our Founding Fathers called divine providence. I was being lifted into some divine space, and it was ecstatic. I remember clearly a visual image I had while sitting there with Dr. Kantor of a shield in front of my heart that was melting. And as the shield melted away, my heart spoke. And I heard it speak in a different way than I'd ever heard before. It was a soft voice. It was the voice of my inner truth, and it felt very undefended—as if I were allowing my inner spirit to speak. It was a very powerful experience, and of course I wanted to come back to his office and do it again, which I was fortunate enough to be able to do.

The Need for More Research into Trauma and Addiction

Caller: The other half of my question is: How is MDMA used in treating alcoholism?

MM: There are no studies going on now—and I don't think there have been—but I think it would be a very good thing to study.

RLM: It would.

AM: We had one person that stopped smoking. We had a couple people that didn't drink caffeine anymore after our study. We had three people go back to work that had not been able to work. So we found a lot of things that could help.

RLM: Yes. Thank you, Annie. We have another caller here. *Welcome to Mind, Body, Health & Politics.* You're on the air.

Caller: Can you discuss the difference between people who cave in under the trauma and those where it passes over them? Have you found the determining factor?

MM: Many people have been asking that question, and nobody really knows the answer. There is quite a lot of research—there is some association to early childhood trauma and later developing PTSD from a dull trauma. There is now some work suggesting genetic factors. I'm sure it has a lot to do with the kind of support the person has, such that we really don't know the answer to that.

RLM: Do we have time for one more question here? We can get one more in here. *Welcome to Mind, Body, Health & Politics,* you're on the air.

Caller: Thank you so much for the program. I wanted to relay to you and to the listening audience that MDMA was really a heart medicine for me. It was as if I came into the realm of pure love. The few people that I was around, I felt safe with. And I saw the beauty in them. I felt the angels were all there. I just came into a realm of pure love.

RLM: Thank you; and that, I think, is what you heard from Annie and Michael.

AM and MM: Yes.

THREE

Psilocybin

Substance: Psilocybin mushrooms (various species), containing the compounds psilocybin, psilocin, and baeocystin

Schedule: I*

Psilocybin mushrooms are mushrooms that naturally contain the psychedelic compounds psilocybin, psilocin, and baeocystin. They are commonly called psychedelic mushrooms, magic mushrooms, and shrooms. After ingesting psilocybin mushrooms, a person might feel any of these effects: a sense of euphoria, alterations in thinking, visualizations (when eyes are open or closed), an altered sense of time, synesthesia (when a sensation or image of a sense is experienced as being other than the sense being stimulated, such as sounds being perceived as colors), and spiritual experiences.[†]

Humans have a long history with psilocybin mushrooms. They are possibly depicted in Stone Age rock art in Europe and Africa, and have a history of use in pre-Columbian Mesoamerica. It is thought that many cultures have used these mushrooms in their religious rites and ceremonies to enhance communion with the divine. However, psi-

---

*No recognized medical use and high potential for abuse.
[†]https://en.wikipedia.org/wiki/Psilocybin_mushroom.

locybin mushrooms have been rejected and suppressed at times: "After the Spanish conquest, Catholic missionaries campaigned against the cultural tradition of the Aztecs, dismissing the Aztecs as idolaters, and the use of hallucinogenic plants and mushrooms, like other pre-Christian traditions, were quickly suppressed. The Spanish believed the mushroom allowed the Aztecs and others to communicate with devils. In converting people to Catholicism, the Spanish pushed for a switch from *teonanácatl* to the Catholic sacrament of the Eucharist. Despite this history, in some remote areas the use of *teonanácatl* has remained."[*]

Psilocybin mushrooms were first mentioned in the medical literature in the London *Medical and Physical Journal* in 1799.[†] The case concerned a man who picked wild-growing *Psilocybe semilanceata* mushrooms and served them to his family.

Interest in and use of mushrooms grew significantly after the mid-to-late 1950s in Europe and America, in part due to the 1957 article in *Life* magazine by R. Gordon Wasson and his wife Valentina, who were thought to be the first Caucasians to participate in an indigenous psilocybin ceremony.[‡] In 1958 Albert Hofmann first identified the active compounds in these mushrooms: psilocybin and psilocin.

Over the next decades, the exploration of entheogens (psychoactive substances that induce spiritual experiences) was promoted by authors Timothy Leary and Terence McKenna, among many others. The availability of psilocybin mushrooms from wild and cultivated sources has made it among the most widely used of the psychedelic

[*]https://en.wikipedia.org/wiki/Psilocybin_mushroom, quoting from Paul Stamets, *Psilocybin Mushrooms of the World* (Berkeley: Ten Speed Press, 1996), 11; and Albert Hofmann, "The Mexican Relatives of LSD," *LSD: My Problem Child* (New York: McGraw-Hill, 1980), 49–71.

[†]E. Brande, "Mr. E. Brande, on a poisonous species of Agaric," *The Medical and Physical Journal* 3 (1799): 41–44.

[‡]R. Gordon Wasson, "Seeking the Magic Mushroom," *Life* (May 13, 1957): 100–120. Available online at http://goo.gl/1Cfhnr.

drugs. Today, the therapeutic effects of this medicine are being explored by scientists.

Breaking the Psychedelic Research Taboo

There aren't many scientists around the world—and certainly not in this country—who have done research on psychedelic medicines, because the United States government has made it extremely difficult to do.

Scientists like Roland Griffiths, PhD, and Katherine MacLean, PhD, of Johns Hopkins University are risking their careers researching psilocybin.

Griffiths is a professor in the departments of psychiatry and neurosciences at the Johns Hopkins University School of Medicine. His research on mood-altering drugs has been largely supported by government grants.

In 1999 he initiated a research program at Johns Hopkins investigating the effects of the classic hallucinogen psilocybin that includes studies of psilocybin-occasioned mystical-type experiences in healthy volunteers, psilocybin-facilitated treatment of psychological distress in cancer patients, psilocybin-facilitated treatment of cigarette smoking cessation, psilocybin effects in beginning and long-term meditators, and psilocybin effects in religious leaders.

As a postdoctoral research fellow and faculty member at the Johns Hopkins University School of Medicine, Katherine MacLean worked with Griffiths and his team. MacLean is the director of the Psychedelic Education and Continuing Care Program and a research scientist at the University of California, Davis. Her research on psilocybin and personality change suggests that this class of medicines may play an important role in enhancing mental health, promoting emotional well-being and creativity throughout the lifespan.

Griffiths and MacLean's groundbreaking research on psilocybin and depression stunned the world and rocked the pharmaceutical industry. We live in a world where research can subject you to various kinds of scrutiny—whether it's from the U.S. government or your own academic colleagues. These two scientists are to be applauded for their research and for bringing the information to us. But let's go back to before 2009, to an unprecedented study that was published in the peer-reviewed journal *Psychopharmacology*.

A Groundbreaking Study

In 2006, Griffiths initiated a research study on psilocybin ("Psilocybin Can Occasion Mystical-type Experiences Having Substantial and Sustained Personal Meaning and Spiritual Significance") that caught the attention of fellow researchers, including Dave Nichols of Purdue University's Department of Medicinal Chemistry and Molecular Pharmacology, who has also been on my radio program and whose research is reported in this book. Here is what Nichols said regarding Griffiths's findings on psilocybin:

> The article by Griffiths et al. in this issue of *Psychopharmacology* should make all scientists interested in human psychopharmacology sit up and take notice. It is the first well-designed, placebo-controlled clinical study in more than four decades to examine the psychological consequences of the effects of the hallucinogenic [psychedelic] agent known as psilocybin. In fact, one would be hard pressed to find a single study of psychedelics from any earlier era that was as well done or as meaningful. Perhaps more importantly, despite the notion by many people that psychedelics are nothing more than troublesome drugs of abuse, the present study convincingly demonstrates that, when used appropriately, these compounds can produce remarkable, possibly beneficial, effects that certainly deserve further study.*

---

*Griffiths et al., "Psilocybin Can Occasion Mystical-type Experiences Having Substantial and Sustained Personal Meaning and Spiritual Significance," *Psychopharmacology* 187 (2006): 268–83.

Also taking note of Griffiths's research was Harriet de Wit of the Department of Psychiatry at the University of Chicago, who said:

> People have long sought meaning and significance in their lives through a variety of spiritual practices including prayer, fasting, chanting, solitude, and meditation. Historically, some of these practices have included the use of certain psychoactive plants. A common theme of these experiences, with or without the aid of psychoactive agents, has been to free oneself of the bounds of everyday perception and thought in a search for universal truths and enlightenment. To a large extent, this type of subjective and uniquely human experience has enjoyed little credibility in the mainstream scientific world and, thus, has been given little scientific attention. However, it may be time now to recognize these extraordinary subjective experiences, even if they are, at present, not directly verifiable by objective measures and even if they sometimes involve claims about ultimate realities that lie outside the purview of science.*

De Wit goes on to say that the article by Griffiths et al. describes one of the first attempts to study these experiences in a systematic scientific investigation. She applauds the study and talks about how it's rigorous, how it includes controlled double-blind administration, and how it was the first study conducted in a specifically designed environment.

Now that we've read about how well-received these studies have been, it's my pleasure to introduce my next interview with the studies' authors, Roland Griffiths and Katherine MacLean.

---

*James MacKillop, and Harriet de Wit (editors), *The Wiley-Blackwell Handbook of Addiction Psychopharmacology* (West Sussex, UK: Wiley-Blackwell, John Wiley & Sons Ltd, 2013).

Spiritual Psychopharmacology

Roland Griffiths, PhD, and Katherine MacLean, PhD

January 16, 2014

ROLAND GRIFFITHS, PhD, is a psychopharmacologist and professor at Johns Hopkins University in the departments of Psychiatry and Neuroscience. Griffiths' psychopharmacology research has been at the cutting-edge of neuroscience for over forty years. He also has a long-term meditation practice. Katherine MacLean, PhD, is an academically trained research scientist and meditation practitioner with a long-standing interest in the brain, consciousness, and the science of well-being. As a graduate student at the University of California, Davis, Katherine was supported by a prestigious National Science Foundation research fellowship to study the effects of intensive meditation training on concentration, emotional well-being, and brain function.

Psilocybin and the Primary Mystical Experience

RLM: Welcome, Roland Griffiths and Katherine MacLean. What's the beginning of the story of this groundbreaking research on psilocybin?

Roland Griffiths, PhD (RG): I'm a psychopharmacologist. I study mood-altering drugs and have been doing so at Johns Hopkins for over forty years. About twenty years ago I took up a meditation practice that opened for me a fascinating window into the nature of spiritual experience, and it got me asking questions about spiritual transformation. I became very intrigued with meditation, the nature of spirituality, and comparative religion in a way that I never had been before.

I was studying mostly drugs of abuse, so there wasn't an immediate connection to psychedelics until I was reminded of the work conducted mostly in the 1950s and 1960s, with a whole class of classic hallucinogens—LSD like serotonergically mediated hallucinogens including LSD, psilocybin, mescaline, and DMT [N,N-dimethyl-tryptamine, the active ingredient in ayahuasca]. There had been at least one very seminal study from the 1960s, the Good Friday Experiment, in which psilocybin was said to have occasioned religious-like experiences in seminary students . . .

RLM: What does that mean when you use words like "religious-like experience" or the word "spirituality"?

RG: [Laughing] Spirituality is one of those words that I use frequently and actually choose not to define. It's like a projective test—people end up talking about whatever their personal thoughts of spirituality are. But I can talk about the primary mystical experience, and that's what our research has largely focused in on. Let me tell you about the setting and condition in which we give psilocybin, and then I'll describe the core of this experience, which also relates to our belief in the potential therapeutic importance of these compounds.

The Gold Standard: Double-Blind with Active Placebo

RG: We administer psilocybin to carefully screened, psychologically and medically healthy volunteers who have been well prepared for the sessions. They meet for at least eight contact clinical hours with two guides or monitors who will be present with them throughout the psilocybin session.

RLM: When did this study take place?

RG: The first study we conducted, in healthy volunteers, was initiated in about the year 1999 and published in 2006. We compared the acute effects of psilocybin with that of an active control drug—in this case it was methylphenidate, or Ritalin.

RLM: An active placebo, in other words?

RG: Yes, under deeply blinded conditions that lead people to believe they could receive any number of different compounds—including psilocybin. Even the guides or monitors were blinded to those drug conditions, so we blinded this as deeply as we could.

RLM: For our listeners, please note we're talking about the importance of having the placebo do something—what's called "active." Otherwise the subjects can obviously tell when they are getting the medicine or the placebo, because if nothing happens then the subject says to themselves, "Oh, I must be in the placebo group." The people who get something and feel something happening say, "Oh, I must be getting the drug." Their understanding of that affects the study. Roland is saying the subjects who were given a placebo were given a feeling, so neither group could tell who was on the actual medicine and who was on a placebo. Right?

RG: Furthermore, in this first group everyone was "hallucinogen-naive." Thus, volunteers could not confidently know whether or not the effects they experienced were due to psilocybin or a range of other psychoactive drugs.

RLM: If that hadn't been the case, immediately they'd say, "Oh yes, this is psilocybin, and I've had this before." Instead, everybody was naive.

Tough but Fair
Passing Johns Hopkins Institutional Review Board

RLM: How long did it take you to get permission to do that study in 1999? How many years prior to that had you been applying for permission and sending in your papers?

RG: Unlike the testimonies you described earlier, we got approval relatively quickly. I would say over the course of a year. We got approval both from the Food and Drug Administration and from the DEA. The biggest hurdle was our institutional review board [IRB] at Hopkins. We were scrutinized much more closely than I've ever been scrutinized for any study—and I've spent my entire career conducting clinical pharmacology studies with various drugs, so I have a lot of experience with approvals at both the institutional level and with the FDA. The initial reluctance to approve this research was understandable in light of the misunderstanding about safety that resulted from the cultural backlash against these compounds in reaction to the widespread, often careless nonmedical use in the 1960s.

RLM: How were you scrutinized?

RG: There was a lot of reluctance. The study was reviewed by our IRB, and it was then sent out for external review, which is unprecedented in my experience. It was reviewed not only by our IRB, but also by administrative authorities within the institution and attorneys within the institution. On several occasions the study was suspended while other new questions were asked and additional reviews were sought. But I'm proud of Johns Hopkins for stepping forward on this. This was the first study to administer a classic hallucinogen to hallucinogen-naive individuals in about thirty years. Johns Hopkins could have taken the institutionally protective position of denying approval. But, instead, they chose science over potential institutional risk. The IRB asked all the right questions and ultimately concluded that the risks did not appear to outweigh the potential benefits. Understandably, they monitored the protocol closely. Now, more than fifteen years later, we have developed a very solid record of safety, having administered psilocybin to over 250 participants in more than five hundred sessions.

Trailblazing for Future Research

RG: We went forward and have actually now seen a sea change in the approvability of such studies. We have published several articles in this area now. Since we were approved, Charles Grob got approved, and other investigators have been approved for psilocybin research. We've written a major safety paper about what kinds of safeguards are needed to conduct these trials. The situation now is vastly different than it was fifteen years ago for academic scientists who would like to initiate this kind of research. They will still be subject to the scrutiny of the DEA and the requirement that the drug be kept under safe conditions. In our case, we already had a Schedule I drug vault.

RLM: You didn't have to build a concrete bunker with a steel plate in the back, surveillance cameras, and bodyguards?

RG: In fact, the pharmacy in our building is under camera control, with security guards that patrol the campus and the buildings. We already fulfilled many of those kinds of requirements.

Scientific Observation of Mystical Experiences

RG: We carefully prepare volunteers who have been screened. On the day of the session they come into a room that is aesthetically attractive—a living room–like situation, where there's a couch and chairs, nice wall hangings, and rugs. The volunteers swallow a psilocybin capsule with water. Psilocybin is the active ingredient in the magic mushroom, but our psilocybin was synthesized by Dave Nichols. Dave Nichols is probably the world's preeminent organic medicinal chemist who has focused his career on understanding the basic pharmacology of hallucinogens. He synthesized the psilocybin, so we are giving the pure compound. Thus, we know exactly what dose we're administering.

People take the capsule and are invited to lie down on the couch—they're encouraged to use eye shades, and headphones through which they listen to a program of music—largely classical, some world music. They are encouraged to direct their attention inward, on their inner experience. We invite them to simply go in and explore, so that the experience is not really "guided." During sessions, two monitors are present, very often right by the participant's couch. The monitors are there to provide support if needed and reassurance about consensual reality should the participant lose bearing of that at the high dose of psilocybin that we administer, which is 30 milligrams per 70 kilograms of body weight. That's about equivalent to 5 grams of dried mushroom of potency—a very high dose of psilocybin. Under these conditions, psilocybin may produce significant alterations in perception: visual, auditory, and tactile. It may also produce marked changes in mood, affect, and thought processes.

More Real than Reality
Unity, Sacredness, Reverence, and Awe

RG: What's most interesting to us is that under the right conditions—when participants are prepared well and feeling safe—they often have experiences that map onto naturally occurring mystical-type experiences. These are experiences that have been reported by mystics and religious figures throughout the ages and have been carefully described throughout the literature of the psychology of religion—very prominently represented by William James in the early 1900s. There have been measures developed for rigorously assessing the phenomenological domains of these transcendent experiences.

The major feature of this experience, endorsed by about 70 percent of our volunteers, is the interconnectedness of all people and things—a sense of unity, that all is one. This is accompanied by a sense of sacredness or reverence, sometimes described as awe. Also, a sense that the experience is more real and true than everyday waking consciousness. The other qualities of the experience are a sense of open-heartedness—sometimes described as love, gratitude, or peacefulness—and a sense of transcendence of time and space, when past and future collapse into the present moment and that's all there is, the present moment. Space becomes boundless and time endless. And then finally, a sense of ineffability. One of the first things people say after having this kind of experience is, "I can't possibly tell you what the experience was about. I can't put it into words because they just don't fit."

A Lasting Change

RG: The remarkable thing is, not only do people endorse that experience immediately after the session, but at a one- or two-month follow-up and more than a year follow-up, they continue to say the experience has positively changed their attitudes about themselves, their lives, and other people. They claim to be more prosocial, more generous, and more loving. People will also claim to make changes in their behavior in accordance with that; so, for instance, they may take up a meditation practice, eat more healthily, or exercise more regularly. Caretaking of self and others emerges from this experience. The experience, of course, is over at the end of the session. But the memory endures, and the principal features—this interconnectedness of all things, sacredness, the sense of the truth value of it, a sense of heart opening, transcendence of time and space, and ineffability—this whole package comes together as the mystical experience.

RLM: When people reflect back on their psilocybin experience, they say their lives are changed in a positive direction. Their core sense of who they are and what they're doing in this world has changed. And they report this a year later?

RG: Yes, more than a year later. And importantly, it is not just the participants who report these changes. In several studies, we have conducted interviews with the participants' friends, family, and colleagues at work. That data converges with the types of changes reported by the volunteers. Furthermore, Katherine did a very interesting study that she may be able to describe to you in which their personality has been shown to be changed.*

Permanent Changes in Personality
Measuring Increases in Openness

Katherine MacLean, PhD (KM): The brief story about personality is that psychologists have come up with a way of categorizing the general tendencies a person has for thinking, feeling, and acting in the world. They've kind of come up with general areas, or factors, in which you can be high, low, or average. One of these areas is openness. People high in openness tend to be creative. It's linked to intelligence, problem solving, being sensitive to your feelings and those of others, being open to new ideas, and being more flexible approaching new situations. We saw an increase in openness after the single psilocybin session with the highest dose. That increase persisted for up to more than a year after the session in the people who had this classic mystical experience. You might have someone who had changes in time and space, but no feeling of sacredness—that wouldn't be the full package. The people who had the full package of mystical experience were still reporting increases in this area of openness a year later.

The measure of personality in psychology is based on a self-reporting survey of two hundred questions, agreeing or disagreeing about whether it describes you. It's their collective response to all of those different openness items scattered throughout the survey.

---

*K. A. MacLean, M. W. Johnson, and R. R. Griffiths, "Mystical Experiences Occasioned by the Hallucinogen Psilocybin Lead to Increases in the Personality Domain of Openness," *Journal of Psychopharmacology* 25, no. 11 (2011): 1453–61.

This is surprising because personalities generally seem to be stable after about the age of thirty, although some researchers think it can change in adulthood after significant life experiences. There is some change that happens in your teen years and when you go to college or leave home and are finding yourself. But by the time you're thirty years old, your personality has solidified somewhat. We saw increases in openness that were larger than you might expect, even over decades of life experience, if you extrapolate a growth curve that people might be on. So it seems fairly permanent in the people that we studied.

Defining Consciousness Expansion

RLM: *Openness* is an interesting word. How did you operationally* define openness, please?

KM: Luckily, we have an entire field called personality psychology that had already operationalized openness for us. Openness has different aspects. One is fantasy, or imagination. Another facet is intellectual curiosity, or ideas—it's essentially problem solving and abstract thinking. Another area is aesthetics—interest in art and music. Another area is called feelings—that sensibility toward your own and others' feelings. Empathy fits in there. There are two others about practical things: Do you like to try new foods? Would you tend to vote liberally or more conservatively on social issues?

RLM: So it's an openness and the sense of expansion, or broadening, of one's experience in life. It's not necessarily openness in terms of, say, transparency and revealing everything about oneself.

KM: Right. That's a good distinction. Openness in our context is more

---

Operationalization is a scientific term meaning the exact manner in which a variable is measured. It identifies one or more specific, observable events or conditions such that any other researcher can independently measure and/or test for them.

broad-mindedness and approaching new situations in a creative and flexible way. It's more of a motivational tendency in terms of which things you seek out and how you respond to new situations.

RLM: Do you think that's why, anecdotally, these substances have been referred to as consciousness expanding?

KM: Anecdotally, it certainly fits with what we're seeing now with this controlled instrument.* Basically, both recreational users and people in the early uncontrolled clinical trials report increases in interest in art and music, creativity, and pursuing things that they wouldn't normally pursue before their experience.

RLM: Katherine, did the subjects in the 30 percent that had difficulties— be it anxiety, panic, and so forth—also have the sense of openness in your study?

KM: Sometimes people would have both anxiety and a mystical experience. In the openness report we made the distinction between those who had a full mystical experience and those who had not, not necessarily those who had anxiety and fear and those who didn't. Some of the people who changed in openness also experienced anxiety and fear.

A Medicine, Not a Drug

KM: The important thing is that we actually meet with people the day after the session. In our current study, for example, we have several meetings with some of the participants after their session. A lot of that is helping people to work through the acute effects and the experiences that they had on the drug and discussing how those may affect their lives in a more holistic way. That piece is also missing during uncontrolled recreational use.

---

*An instrument is a tool used for measurement, in this case the survey.

RLM: One of the takeaways for our listeners is that if they were to take this medicine as a recreational drug rather than a medicine, under these properly controlled conditions, they stand about a one-in-three chance of having a negative experience.

RG: Possibly higher. One of three is under our optimized conditions in which people are really well screened and well prepared.

KM: This was an increase in people who were already high in openness, but also psychologically healthy and well educated. There is a particular demographic that shows this increase. It's possible that you could have increases in openness without a stable foundation that would not be beneficial. Just being higher in openness is not necessarily a good thing.

It's important to understand the context of the research—any of the benefits that we're seeing are restricted to the sample that we studied. This is why we're excited to expand into other patient populations and demographics to see, again, what the balance of benefit and risk is.

Fear and Trembling
The Window into Inner Self

Evangelizing the Psychedelic Experience

RLM: Do people become evangelical about this medicine after their mystical experiences? I would think they would.

RG: Interestingly, no. We have administered the drug under very well-prepared and sacramental conditions—or conditions that approach sacramental views. It's an experience that most participants hold dearly to themselves. They believe the research is important and what they participated in is as important as anything that they have done.

RLM: Exactly. That's what makes me think they'd want to go out and say to their friends and family, "Hey, you've got to get a hold of some of this stuff," [laughing] because that's how human beings are. If you go to the store and get something good, you go tell your friends, right?

RG: Yes, but that doesn't necessarily follow, because we know that if people take high doses of psilocybin mushrooms, some will have remarkable experiences, but other people will have terrible, sometimes traumatic experiences. Some people are going to be thrown into harm's way because of fear or panic or anxiety, which is not uncommon even under our conditions. Even in our studies, about 30 percent of people will endorse having experiences of great fear or anxiety, sometimes as fearful as anything that they've ever experienced.

So there is an important footnote to this—that even giving psilocybin to highly screened participants under optimized conditions, after hours of preparation, with two people sitting at their side, we still have a 30 percent probability that they're going to experience extraordinary anxiety. But we know that under conditions in which people are not carefully monitored or selected, some people end up panicking—reacting to that fear. Under uncontrolled conditions, some people end up running out into traffic or doing harm to themselves. Others will report enduring psychological problems that last for years after some experiences.

RLM: Not your subjects.

RG: No. None of our subjects did. We know we can do this safely under appropriate conditions.

Fear Can Lead to Transcendence

RLM: Let's stay with your subjects who got anxiety, both directly after the initial administration and then also that same group a year later—how did they look back on that anxiety and panic? What was their take on it?

RG: It's a great question, Richard, and we actually don't have the power to tease apart the long-term impact. I can just tell you anecdotally that it is really variable across volunteers. Some will have an extraordinary sense of panic that will then actually open up into transcendence.

RLM: That's the reason I'm asking.

RG: Fear sometimes becomes a doorway opening to an experience of transcendence. We do have a smaller percentage of people who get caught in the classic "bad trip," during which they experience anxiety or dysphoric struggle for most of the session. The important thing about those people in our studies is that none of them felt that they had been harmed by that experience.

RLM: That matches an interview I did recently, Roland, of a man who took a psychedelic medicine, and for five and a half hours he was screaming and yelling—anxious and panicked—and when I interviewed him the next day he said, "Yeah, the people around me thought it was terrible, but I felt like I was going through something very important, and I have no regrets about it whatsoever. In fact, I feel like I mastered the anxiety by going through it, getting into it, and then coming out of it."

RG: Yes. Under these conditions, when these challenging experiences can be supported well, participants often feel that it's a growth experience. However, there are people who would say, "I would never, ever, ever want to have that experience again."

RLM: [Laughing] It sounds very similar to patients of mine who are not taking any psychedelic medicine, but who have anxiety and panic. When we go through it together, and they learn tools for dealing with it, they then have a sense of mastery. They don't want to call the anxiety and panic a good thing, but the fact that they now have a sense of mastery and confidence over it is a good thing. They are no longer fearful of it happening again.

Taking Psilocybin Seriously: Medicine or Drug?

Risks of Recreational Use

RLM: Maybe there are some examples of people—I don't know of any on record—walking into traffic. Do you actually know of an example of that, Roland?

RG: Yes, unfortunately I do. People jumping off of cliffs and off of buildings . . .

RLM: You have examples of that?

RG: Yes . . . absolutely.

RLM: Well, caveat emptor, folks who are listening. Very much so.

RG: Yes, this underscores the risk of taking these compounds under conditions in which one is not optimally supported, and a lot of recreational use occurs under those conditions.

RLM: The way I differentiate that, Roland, is that what you're doing is administering a medicine, and when people take it on their own, they're taking a drug. One is called drug use and the other is called taking a medicine under proper protocol and conditions.

Psychedelic Medicines as Psychological Surgery

KM: One analogy is the idea of going in for a surgery, except the potential risks and benefits with the psychedelic experience are psychological not physical. For a surgery, you might have a huge potential benefit, but certain risks may come up acutely during the surgery, and it's not something that you would want to necessarily undertake on your own. [RLM laughs] You want the right kind of medical safety, and the experts who can guide you through those potentially risky scenarios. And then you want to follow up afterward, to make sure that the risks, if there were any lingering effects, have been minimized. It's not a perfect analogy, but it makes sense when people are thinking, "Why would you ever want to go through something where there is risk involved?" It's a matter of balancing the potential benefits with the acute risks of cognitively working through the experience that you've had.

RLM: I think that's a great analogy actually, Katherine. Anybody can just grasp on to that and say, "Sure, I would let a surgeon cut open my stomach and go inside and do some work, but I'm sure not going to sit at home and cut open my stomach." It's a dramatic but great example of saying, "Yes, this is a very powerful medicine, and used under proper conditions it is a medicine, but take it home and you might be cutting your stomach open and having to deal with anxiety and panic on your own."

Current Research for Cancer Insight

RLM: Roland, you've got one minute to tell us about the cancer study at Johns Hopkins.

RG: We have recently completed a study in cancer patients who are experiencing anxiety or depression because of a cancer diagnosis. Cancer -Insight.org provides the information.* The results, along with results from a similar study conducted at New York University, appear very promising. These studies are currently under review for publication.

RLM: We're going to have to wrap up. I thank you both very much for taking the time from your busy lives to present this information, and I hope I have the opportunity to have you both on the program again in the future.

---

*"The Johns Hopkins Psilocybin Research Project study team is pleased to report that enrollment for this study has now been completed. We are optimistic about initiating a follow-up study in cancer patients in 2017."

•••

Friday Night Meeting with Charlie Grob

My next interview on psilocybin is with Charlie Grob, MD, with whom we talked in chapter 2 about his work on MDMA. As I mentioned in chapter 2, I had the privilege of first meeting Charlie Grob at my home in the early 1990s, during something called the "Friday night meetings." These monthly meetings were an opportunity for researchers in the psychedelic community from far and wide to socialize and share ideas. It is a great honor to include the second part of his interview.

Seeking Solace for the Terminally Ill

Charles Grob, MD

Excerpt from November 29, 2011

CHARLES S. GROB, MD, is the director of the Division of Child and Adolescent Psychiatry at Harbor-UCLA Medical Center and Professor of Psychiatry and Pediatrics at the UCLA School of Medicine. In the early 1990s he conducted the first government-approved psychobiological research study of MDMA (see chapter 2), and he was the principal investigator of an international research project in the Brazilian Amazon studying ayahuasca (see chapter 4). He has also completed an investigation of the safety and efficacy of psilocybin treatment in advanced-cancer patients with anxiety and published his findings in the January 2011 issue of the *Archives of General Psychiatry*. He is the editor of *Hallucinogens: A Reader* (2002) and the coeditor (with Roger Walsh) of *Higher Wisdom: Eminent Elders Explore the Continuing Impact of Psychedelics* (2005). He is a founding board member of the Heffter Research Institute.

Harbor-UCLA Medical Center
Revives Psilocybin Research

RLM: You have been doing research on psilocybin down at Harbor-UCLA Medical Center with cancer patients for some time, and we would very much like to hear about it.

Charles Grob, MD (CG): We received permission from the FDA and other regulatory agencies to conduct a protocol we had written, which would allow us to utilize a psilocybin treatment model for individuals with advanced cancer and anxiety. The primary target symptoms would be the anxiety—not the cancer per se. These studies were inspired by the early researchers, starting in the late '50s with Eric Kast and then into the '60s with Sidney Cohen* and Gary Fisher. Tremendous work was done by Walter Pahnke† and Stanislav Grof, when they utilized the prototype classic hallucinogen LSD to treat terminal cancer patients, reporting remarkable improvements in psychologic status and also reduced perception of pain and need for narcotic pain medication.

I had dreamed of doing this study for decades, since I first read Grof's work. I had seen him give a talk in New York City in the early '70s. That in and of itself was an inspiration for me to get my credentials so I could work in this field.

Study Results Published in
a Mainstream Scientific Journal

CG: In the early 2000s, we were the first group since the late '60s given permission to work with a hallucinogenic treatment model

---

*Steven J. Novak, "LSD before Leary: Sidney Cohen's Critique of 1950s Psychedelic Drug Research," *Isis* 88, no. 1 (March 1997): 87–110.
†Walter Pahnke designed the 1962 Marsh Chapel Experiment, also called the "Good Friday Experiment," investigating the effects of psilocybin on religiously predisposed subjects.

in advanced-stage cancer patients. Beginning in 2004 we treated twelve individuals in a double-blind placebo control model, where each subject functions as their own control. Following a very thorough screening and preparation process, each of the subjects came in for two separate sessions. Some of the subjects received psilocybin first and placebo second, others the other way around. But it was all blinded, meaning neither the subjects, nor myself, nor my staff knew what they were getting on any one occasion. They would get either one or the other; though generally we could figure it out.

Essentially, our twelve subjects did very well. I should say first and foremost there were no adverse effects—no one had a bad trip, severe anxiety, or a paranoid reaction. People tolerated the experience very well. I'll say also that my two research coordinators, Marycie Hagerty and Alicia Danforth, and I prepared our subjects very well for the experience. We met and spoke with them on a number of occasions, helping them understand the range of experiences that might occur. We sat with them for the full six hours of the experience and did all of the treatments on weekends. Following treatment, we provided help with integrating the experience, and we remained in touch for the six-month data follow-up; we were with many of our subjects for the remaining time of their lives.

RLM: What was the dose that they got?

CG: They got 0.2 milligrams per kilogram of body weight of pure synthetic psilocybin.* That would be a moderate dose level, and subjects tolerated it well—there were no safety issues. We saw some indices of anxiety improve over time, we saw some indication that mood improved, and overall there was an improved quality of life.

Our results, I think, were of sufficient interest—as well as the fact that we were doing this first study in many decades was of sufficient

---

*This dose represents less than half of the dose that occasioned fearful responses in many subjects in Griffiths and MacLean's work.

interest—that our manuscript reviewing the study and our findings was published in the January 2011 issue of the *Archives of General Psychiatry*. The *Archives of General Psychiatry* is generally considered to be the number one impact journal in the whole field of psychiatry, so we were pleased to get validation by the mainstream in our field. This provided an opportunity for colleagues who may not have been aware of what we were doing to read about this work. After we conducted our investigation, two other research groups in the country got permission and are now running their own studies using psilocybin to treat advanced-cancer anxiety.

The Active Placebo
Manufacturing a Psychedelish Experience

RLM: Did you use an active or inactive placebo?

CG: We used an active placebo and decided to model it along the lines of what some of the studies from the '60s used. We used niacin [vitamin B₃]. I'm not sure I would use niacin again, but we did want to induce some kind of response so the individual knew that they were on a compound. Niacin has its own range of effects that we thought were distracting from what we were trying to do, so for follow-up studies we will probably use a different placebo.

The Future of Psilocybin Research
Finding Funding for New Studies

RLM: What about the future of your research with psilocybin?

CG: There are studies at Johns Hopkins with Roland Griffiths and at NYU with Stephen Ross. We're very pleased that this field is starting to move forward once again, and these are two very reputable research groups. I should also mention that the funding and the encouragement and help with development of the protocol came from the Heffter Research Institute, which is another not-for-profit foundation that is focused on helping to develop, facilitate, and find funding for future studies looking at the range of effects of hallucinogens in humans. And again, Heffter is also challenged with the whole funding issue—that's been an enormous obstacle for the field.

If we get funding, we'll submit a new protocol to the regulatory agencies, asking to work with additional patients who have advanced medical illness. We would like to make a couple of changes from our original protocol, which would include a slightly higher dose and the opportunity for a second follow-up or booster session. All of our subjects had the same recommendation at the end of their treatment: that an opportunity be created in future protocols for a second follow-up session. They felt this would be of great value to the challenging life circumstances that they were going through.

Going Organic

RLM: We do have a call. Welcome to *Mind, Body, Health & Politics*, you're on the air.

Caller: Why do they use a synthetic instead of an organic compound?

RLM: Great question. Is that accurate?

CG: That is. There are two reasons. One is to minimize variability. You want a consistent dosage of the alkaloid to be present, and you may see varying levels of the active alkaloids from one batch of mushrooms to the next. The other reason really gets back to the fact that our medical system and the FDA are much more comfortable dealing with synthetic compounds rather than whole plant products. There might be a therapeutic advantage to one day looking at the actual mushroom. Whereas our study just utilizes one alkaloid, psilocybin, which breaks down to another alkaloid, psilocin, in the body, the actual mushrooms contain a combination of psilocybin, psilocin, and baeocystin. The contribution of baeocystin to the psychotropic effect would be interesting to study. Those investigations are an awfully long way into the future.

The Retreat Model of
Psychedelic-Assisted Psychotherapy

RLM: Regarding psilocybin for psychotherapeutic purposes in the therapist's office: Do we have a future? Does it look like we are going to live long enough to see it, Charles, or is that too far into the future for us?

CG: It's hard to imagine a treatment model that could be transportable and utilized in any setting. We're not going to be able to write out a prescription and tell someone to have this experience and come back and report. That's not going to happen.

The most viable model I can think of is what Albert Hofmann suggested, which is retreat/treatment centers where individuals who have been trained and certified to conduct this kind of work would work with individuals to prepare them, sit with them, guide them through the terrain, and help integrate the process afterward. With many medical and surgical procedures, not just any surgeon or internist can conduct particular procedures. They first have to get trained and certified so that they have adequate training and can adhere to the necessary safety parameters. Something along the same lines will probably be done in this area.

I don't know whether we will be around to see it. We've already waited a long time. Progress has been minimal, although I'm hopeful that the last two years are an indication that progress will be picking up in the near future.

●●●

Globally, there are so few scientists conducting research into psychedelic substances that most of them know one another personally, and they are well aware of each other's contributions to the growing body of knowledge. Over the decades the extraordinarily courageous, groundbreaking work of Countess Amanda Feilding and her colleague David Nutt has come to us from England, whose attitudes and laws are easily as narrow and draconian as ours.

Psilocybin and Depression
Amanda Feilding
Excerpt from July 7, 2016

AMANDA FEILDING is an English artist, scientist, and drug-policy reformer. In 1998 Amanda founded the Beckley Foundation, a charitable trust that promotes a rational, evidence-based approach to global drug policy and initiates, designs, and carries out pioneering neuroscientific and clinical research into the effects of psychoactive substances on the brain and on cognition. She is dedicated to investigating novel treatment pathways for mental and physical conditions as well as developing new means to enhance creativity and well-being.

When Nothing Else Has Worked
Psilocybin Provides Longer-term Improvement for Depression

Amanda Feilding (AF): We've just recently done the first study using psilocybin in the treatment of chronic depression. This was just a small pilot study, but it showed that 67 percent of participants, who had been depressed for eighteen years on average and had been unresponsive to every other form of treatment, experienced significant improvement in their symptoms one week later. Three months later 42 percent remained depression free. This is a remarkably high success rate.

RLM: You did pre- and post-testing on these people who were suffering from depression. After the pretesting, what did you administer?

AF: Psilocybin in this case.

RLM: In this case we're talking about psilocybin, another mind-altering substance. Please tell us more about psilocybin and educate us.

AF: Psilocybin is the psychoactive compound in magic mushrooms, that is, the mushrooms that have been used throughout history by shamans and medicine men and women around the world to alter consciousness, bring about revelations or spiritual experiences, and heal people. It wasn't until recently that people in the West knew about these psychoactive mushrooms—largely as a result of amateur mycologist Gordon Wasson's explorations. Traditional societies, particularly in Mexico, have known about the psychedelic properties of magic mushrooms for thousands of years. Albert Hofmann, the discoverer of LSD, synthesized the first psilocybin in 1957.

Albert was an amazing, creative scientist of the highest order. I think Bart Huges was another creative genius, in visualizing the mechanisms underlying the consciousness brought about by psychoactive substances and other techniques. Bart wasn't totally right all the way through, but it's remarkable how much of what he projected is turning out to be the reality.

No Need for Mushrooms

RLM: Albert Hofmann who synthesized LSD also synthesized psilocybin.

AF: Yes.

RLM: Now we actually have a product that can be made rather than necessarily hunting for the mushrooms. Did psilocybin become illegal in England as well?

AF: Yes, mushrooms became illegal quite recently. It was a crazy thing: little old ladies who pick mushrooms in the countryside are actually criminals! Luckily no one really knows the word "psilocybin." This makes it easier to do scientific research with psilocybin than with LSD, which are probably the three most toxic letters in the world. Sad, because actually LSD is an incredible compound that can bring enormous healing powers to our struggling species. I'm hoping that through the very best research we will slowly demonstrate how we can use these compounds to the benefit of the individual, and indeed society.

RLM: Psilocybin has been illegal here in this country for decades. Only recently has some research been allowed. I'm sure you're familiar with the research that Roland Griffiths started.

AF: Absolutely. I worked with him.

RLM: At Johns Hopkins University? You worked with him?

AF: Yes. I worked with him on the study using psilocybin as an aid to psychotherapy in overcoming nicotine addiction. It had an amazingly high success rate of 80 percent.

RLM: Please, tell us a little bit about that study. Describe it for us.

AF: We started it years ago on almost no funding. Basically, they have a wonderful team at Johns Hopkins. They gave two high doses of psilocybin, having prepared the participants very carefully for the occasion. Then basically the participants lie in a comfortable position, with headphones on and eye masks, and get into their inner space. Interestingly, the ones who experienced the most mystical experiences are the ones who had the most successful outcomes. They had a very high success rate, with 80 percent of the participants continuing to abstain from smoking for six months or more. Now, there's an enlarged study being carried out with a brain-imaging component included in the study.

RLM: Regarding the study on depression that Roland did, which you worked on, as I recall, the researchers administered psilocybin one time, and a year later there were still positive results.

AF: I think he's only just completed a study of psilocybin for depression and anxiety in cancer patients, and I wasn't involved in that. Our study at the Beckley/Imperial program was the first to investigate psilocybin's effect on depression. Johns Hopkins is also doing a very interesting study with psilocybin and alcohol addiction.

RLM: In your study with depression and psilocybin, you said that these people were depressed for eighteen years.

AF: On average, yes.

RLM: On average. And 67 percent of them were depression free one week after treatment, and 42 percent of them were in remission three months later?

AF: Yes.

RLM: This is quite remarkable.

AF: Yeah, I think it's one of the highest rates of success that has been recorded. Recently some research with ketamine was done, but it didn't have such a high rate of success, and ketamine has some negative properties, limiting its usefulness as a depression medication.

More Effective with Fewer Doses

RLM: In this country, people are given various kinds of medicines for depression, often including SSRIs, the selective serotonin reuptake inhibitors, because of the effect of serotonin, or the hypothesized effect of serotonin, on depression. What people have to do here is they have to take these medicines 365 days a year. It's basically an annuity for the pharmaceutical companies. The people are buying these medicines, 365 doses a year. Here your study is indicating that people took psilocybin medicine twice, seven days apart, and then had a 42 percent remission in three months, which would indicate that it would be possible to take the medicine maybe four times a year, rather than 365 times a year?

AF: Absolutely.

RLM: This is just with an initial study.

AF: Exactly that. Also, there's a lot of other measures that include general optimism and mindfulness. The participants in our study had been resistant to everything that had been offered to them. I think there's approximately 20 percent of people like this, who don't respond to any treatment, including things like electric shock treatment, which is rather frightening.

RLM: Frightening indeed.

Deep Healing

AF: The people in our study were from that 20 percent. People who hadn't responded to anything previously, and 42 percent were still in remission after three months. As you say, it's four treatments a year. This is what is, in a way, so criminal. If only this approach to healing had been researched over the last fifty years, these people wouldn't need to be suffering, because there would be treatment available. Let's hope that now research will go on to make psychedelic-assisted therapy available. I think it's an amazing new way of getting to the root of the trauma and bringing about a deep healing experience.

•••

Having worked with my share of patients suffering from treatment-resistant depression over the past fifty years, it is bittersweet to share this information about the efficacy of these medicines, which are referred to as psychedelic and therefore kept from the public. It is bitter because—being denied access—the public is forced to the black market whose products are untrustworthy and therefore dangerous. It is sweet because we are finally seeing the results, from around the world, of what psychedelic medicines can do for us.

FOUR

Ayahuasca

Teacher Plant

Substance: Ayahuasca, aka yagé or hoasca

Active Compound(s): N,N-dimethyltryptamine and *Banisteriopsis caapi* as a monoamine oxidase inhibitor (MAOI)

Schedule: I*

Sharing Ideas with a Pioneering Researcher

My first interview about ayahuasca is with Dr. Charlie Grob, with whom we talked in chapters 2 and 3 about his work on MDMA and psilocybin. As I mentioned in those chapters, I had the privilege of first meeting Charlie Grob at my home in the early 1990s, during something called the "Friday night meetings." These monthly meetings were an opportunity for the very small number of brave researchers in the psychedelic community, from far and wide, to socialize and share ideas. You might think of it as a miniconference. It is a great honor to include the third and final part of his interview.

---

*No recognized medical use and high potential for abuse.

Hard Science in the Amazon
Charles Grob, MD
Excerpt from November 29, 2011

CHARLES S. GROB, MD, is director of the Division of Child and Adolescent Psychiatry at Harbor-UCLA Medical Center and Professor of Psychiatry and Pediatrics at the UCLA School of Medicine. In the early 1990s he conducted the first government-approved psychobiological research study of MDMA (see chapter 2) and was the principal investigator of an international research project in the Brazilian Amazon studying ayahuasca. He has also completed an investigation of the safety and efficacy of psilocybin treatment in advanced-cancer patients with anxiety and published his findings in the January 2011 issue of the *Archives of General Psychiatry* (see chapter 3). He is the editor of *Hallucinogens: A Reader* (2002) and the coeditor (with Roger Walsh) of *Higher Wisdom: Eminent Elders Explore the Continuing Impact of Psychedelics* (2005). He is a founding board member of the Heffter Research Institute.

Therapeutic Properties of Ayahuasca

RLM: You went down to the Brazilian Amazon and studied ayahuasca. What can you tell us about its potential use in psychotherapy?

Charles Grob, MD (CG): Ayahuasca is a fascinating compound. It's a decoction* of two plants that grow in the Amazon. Nothing happens when either plant is taken by itself, but when the two plants are brewed together and ingested, a very powerful four-hour altered state experience ensues.

I went down to Brazil with my friend and colleague Dennis McKenna, the ethnobotanist who had established a liaison with the União

---

*Decoction is a method of extraction by boiling herbal or plant material—including stems, roots, bark, and rhizomes—to dissolve the chemicals from the plant.

do Vegetal [UDV]—one of the legal Brazilian syncretic ayahuasca churches down there that's had permission from the government since the mid '80s to utilize ayahuasca as a psychoactive sacrament—but only for their religious ceremonies. It's never used for recreational purposes.

We conducted, in many respects, a state-of-the-art study under very challenging conditions in the Amazon, in the city of Manaus. We had each of the fifteen subjects recruited at random from the UDV. They had to be members for at least ten years. We examined basic physiologic parameters like heart rate, blood pressure, electrocardiogram, and pupillary diameter. We used indwelling intravenous catheters, and we took blood samples out every thirty minutes for pharmacokinetics assessment on and analyses of neuroendocrine secretion. We also did structured psychiatric diagnostic interviews. For the psychiatric assessment, we used matched control populations that had never taken ayahuasca, and then we did diagnostic interviews. I did open-ended life-story interviews. We did neuropsychological testing. We did personality testing. And we got some very interesting results.

First and foremost, the subjects in the ayahuasca religion—part of the UDV—were very high-functioning individuals. They were very impressive. Whereas some of them had significant history of psychopathology prior to their entry into the UDV, it all had appeared to remit. This included severe alcohol and drug addiction. It included severe history of mood disturbance and antisocial behaviors. These individuals, over their time in this religion where they ingested ayahuasca in group ritual context at least twice monthly, had seemingly transformed.

U.S. Supreme Court Rules
Ayahuasca Is Legal for Church Members

RLM: Tell the listeners again what the UDV is.

CG: União do Vegetal translates as Union of the Plants in Portuguese.

It's the name of this religion that came into being approximately sixty years ago. It was founded by a man named Mestre Gabriel, who had interacted with indigenous people in the deep Amazon rainforest in the 1940s while working as a rubber tapper. He discovered the use of ayahuasca, came back to an urban center in eastern Brazil, and developed the structure for a religion that utilized ayahuasca as a psychoactive sacrament. The UDV was illegal from its formation in the early '60s until the mid '80s, when their use of ayahuasca as a ceremonial sacrament was sanctioned under law.

So it's legal in Brazil. I should also mention that subsequently a branch of the UDV was established in Santa Fe, New Mexico, and a few other cities around the United States. They were shut down in the late '90s by U.S. Customs and the DEA. The UDV filed a formal protest that their freedom of religion rights had been violated, so the case went to federal court in New Mexico. I was the expert medical witness for the UDV, so I was very involved in the case. To my surprise the Republican conservative federal judge ruled on behalf of the UDV, agreeing that their freedom of religion rights had been violated and also that the government had not made a successful case as to the relative dangers of ayahuasca to human users.

The Justice Department appealed the decision, and it went to the panel for the Circuit Court of Appeals in Denver. It ruled two to one in favor of the UDV. Then it was appealed again and went to the full appeals court, which ruled nine to five on behalf of the UDV. Then it was appealed *again* and went to the full U.S. Supreme Court in February 2006. Chief Justice John Roberts wrote his first decision as Chief Justice, and he wrote for a unanimous majority. Actually, the court voted unanimously to support the defense of the freedom of religion of the UDV. In that case, at least, it was interesting to see that freedom of religion trumps the drug war.

RLM: What are the practical implications of that Supreme Court decision in terms of people being part of that church?

CG: There are only a few hundred members of the UDV in the United States—in Santa Fe and a few other cities—and I believe the decision literally pertains only to the UDV. There is a second ayahuasca religion from Brazil, the Santo Daime, which is in a few places around the country. But the strict interpretation of the original Supreme Court decision is that it simply addresses members of the UDV and is not a blanket sanction for ayahuasca use.*

Despite Impressive Results, No Research in the United States

RLM: Tell us a bit more about your view on ayahuasca's potential as a psychotherapeutic agent.

CG: Well, it's a fascinating compound. I was really impressed when I was down in Brazil. Subsequently I've met other people and have interviewed individuals who had led very disreputable lives—had a lot of psychopathology, often with very severe alcohol abuse or drug abuse or serious antisocial behavior—and they had in some way or another found their way to this ayahuasca religion. They started to participate in these group ceremonies and had profound psychospiritual epiphanies that led to dramatic transformations of their personality and their conduct. Many of them had gone from functioning on a very marginal level to being pillars of the community.

The UDV members that I met and interacted with in Brazil and in the United States—and I did spend quite a bit of time with them back in the '90s and early 2000s—were very impressive individuals.

I felt there was a great potential to utilize ayahuasca as part of a treatment program for severe alcoholism and drug abuse. I should mention that there is one long-standing clinic in the Peruvian Amazon

---

*In 2009 Santo Daime won the legal right in Oregon to conduct their ceremonies—a decision that was upheld in 2012.

at Tarapoto—the Takiwasi clinic run by a French physician Jacques Mabit—that for some thirty years has been treating Peruvian coca paste addicts. These are individuals who've become quite addicted to a commonly distributed form of the coca plant, or an intermediary product between coca and cocaine, that's highly addictive and in quite widespread use in poor communities in Peru. They've had a very interesting and seemingly functional and longstanding treatment center in Peru.

I've been hoping for some time that it would be possible to conduct a study along those lines in the United States, but there have been no studies conducted as yet on ayahuasca in the United States. The only studies have been from outside the United States. There have been the Brazilian studies* and also some important work coming out of a laboratory at the University of Barcelona in Spain.†

Also recently there have been some efforts in British Columbia to start an ayahuasca treatment program for drug addiction. However, it seems that at this point in time, those efforts may have stalled out through concern from authorities that this is an unscheduled compound. So the future of that program is still up in the air.

Bottom Line: Funding Needed

RLM: Is the main reason that there has been no research on ayahuasca in the United States a matter of funding or is it still political?

CG: Funding. I think there's some antipathy toward looking at plant products, and here you have a combination of two different plants—one of which is highly hallucinogenic. There's been no formal policy

---

*Arran Frood, "Ayahuasca Psychedelic Tested for Depression: A Pilot Study with the Shamanic Brew Hints at Its Therapeutic Potential," ScientificAmerican.com, April 8, 2016, https://www.scientificamerican.com/article/ayahuasca-psychedelic-tested-for -depression/ (accessed April 30, 2017).
†J. Riba and M. J. Barbanoj, "Bringing Ayahuasca to the Clinical Research Laboratory," *Journal of Psychoactive Drugs* 37, no. 2 (2005): 219–30.

decision made. There have only been limited applications to conduct studies, and I'm aware of only one new program that's going forward from a very reputable academic-based research program that might have some greater level of success. If that's the case, I think that could open this field up. Even with the regulatory agencies being more or less amenable to approving well-thought-out studies and making sure that sufficient attention is given to safety, funding is your biggest limitation. Studies are fairly pricey, and private moneys are minimal these days.

•••

An Immediate Connection with a Fellow Psychonaut

When the American ethnopharmacologist, research pharmacognosist, lecturer, and author Dennis McKenna came to visit us at Wilbur Hot Springs, California, for the first time, I felt as though a lifelong family member had just dropped in. It was friendship at first sight with the man who had explored the depths of the Amazon and the depths of his mind at one and the same time.

McKenna is a founding board member and the director of ethnopharmacology at the Heffter Research Institute, a nonprofit organization concerned with the investigation of the potential therapeutic uses of psychedelic medicines. I'm grateful to have had a chance to do the following interview with him about his work with ayahuasca.

Plants Meet People
Dennis McKenna, PhD
September 20, 2011

DENNIS McKENNA, PhD, is an ethnopharmacologist who has studied plant hallucinogens for over forty years. Outside of scientific circles he is best known as the brother of Terence McKenna, a cultural icon in the psychedelic community. Together they are coauthors of *The Invisible Landscape: Mind, Hallucinogens, and the I Ching* and *Psilocybin: Magic Mushroom Grower's Guide—A Handbook for Psilocybin Enthusiasts.* He is also the author of a memoir, *Brotherhood of the Screaming Abyss: My Life with Terence McKenna,* published in 2012.

A North American in a South American Paradigm
The Scientific Responsibilities of an Ethnobotanist

RLM: Tell us some personal experiences, please. How many times do you think you've taken ayahuasca in your lifetime?

Dennis McKenna, PhD (DM): I don't really keep count—I've taken it many times.

RLM: More than one hundred?

DM: I am sure. But I've been working with it for thirty years, and for an ethnobotanist working in the field, it's pretty much impossible not to take it—nor would it even be scientifically responsible not to take it. This is participant observation-type anthropology—if you want to understand how to use it in the indigenous context, you have to get down with the people that are using it and use it with them. You have to look through their lens and join the kinds of realities that it opens up to you. My experience with ayahuasca has been both professional and personal. I went to South America back in the '80s as a graduate student at the University of British Columbia with the objective of approaching this in a rigorous fashion—looking at the chemistry and pharmacology of ayahuasca and the plants used to produce it. That was the subject of my thesis.*

---

*D. J. McKenna, G. H. N. Towers, and F. S. Abbott, "Monoamine Oxidase Inhibitors in South American Hallucinogenic Plants: Tryptamine and ß-carboline Constituents of Ayahuasca," *Journal of Ethnopharmacology* 10, no. 2 (1984): 195–223.

Vomiting: The Safeguard against Overdosing

RLM: Can you overdose on ayahuasca?

DM: It's difficult to do that. There may be a lethal dose but you'd be hard pressed to consume it. You've got your own built-in safeguard, which is that it causes you to vomit. You couldn't possibly keep down a toxic dose of ayahuasca. These medicines are not toxic to the system. In general, the concern is more about the psychological effect, and that you can control—with the right kind of preparation and the right set and setting. You're deliberately inducing an altered state. The question is, "What do you do with that state?" That's where shamanism comes in. They deliberately induce altered states and use that as an opportunity for healing. So that's what we have to learn from shamanism if we're going to ever do this right in biomedicine.

Mind-Body Medicine
The Hoasca Study

DM: I spent time in South America. I collected many samples and analyzed those in the lab and published the results. And then, almost ten years later with some other colleagues, I initiated this biomedical study of ayahuasca with one of the Brazilian churches—what's been called the Hoasca Study. They call it *hoasca*, not *ayahuasca*, in Portuguese. This was probably the most extensive study to date on the possible therapeutic uses of ayahuasca. They use it in a religious context, but there is no doubt that many of the volunteers we interviewed felt it was very important in curing them of their dysfunctional issues—usually either alcoholism or other addictions, but other kinds of what you might call "diseases of the spirit" as well. There is no doubt, in that supporting context, that ayahuasca was beneficial for these people.

RLM: It improved their mind-body health?

DM: Virtually all of them in our study section were in a bad place when they joined the church. They would usually join the UDV at the urging of a friend, because they were having domestic problems, or addiction problems, or they were getting into trouble with the law. They were in a dysfunctional place—not a spiritually balanced place. They felt their ayahuasca experience was what saved them, in the context of the church's supportive environment where there is opportunity for integration and processing of the experience among the members. They often felt that it turned their lives around as long as they stayed on the straight and narrow—which meant taking ayahuasca regularly and staying in the church.

RLM: How regularly?

DM: Their practice is once every two weeks. That's just how they do it, and that's probably about right.

RLM: So we're talking about a therapeutic dose twenty-six times a year roughly to stay on what you call the "straight and narrow."

Not for Everyone

RLM: I heard something you said, and I saw it underlined in red before me, and that was "processing of the experience after the experience." That sounded very important when you said it.

DM: It's very important, and it is an aspect of psychedelic medicine that you don't get with other medicines, even psychopharmaceuticals. Biomedicine these days is pretty much about psychopharmaceuticals. We have a whole pharmacopoeia of these things. There's rarely any follow-up.

RLM: "Go home. Take this every single day, and I'll see you in a month for fifteen minutes."

DM: You can't say that with psychedelics. You can't say, "Take two of these LSD tablets and call me in the morning." I mean . . . you could say that—and I guarantee you, you're going to get a call in the morning. But seriously, you cannot separate these substances' therapeutic use from the context—whether it is a shamanic context, or a psychotherapeutic context, or some combination of those. You have to have a supportive context. Timothy Leary, Ralph Metzner, and the others were absolutely right when they emphasized set and setting. The important thing is that the setting is chosen carefully—that it's a safe environment where you won't be distracted. Whether it's a shaman's hut in the Amazon, or in a clinic, or on top of a mountain; those are the key variables. It's also important to be clear about why you are doing it and what you bring to the table. That is set—your intention. Is it therapeutic? Is it just a learning experience? Is it recreational? All of these are legitimate reasons, but it's important to be clear about the reason for taking it.

RLM: Do we know enough about how to determine who is a candidate for this kind of experience?

DM: If you want to be in an FDA-approved clinical study, then you will be thoroughly screened. They have a protocol to evaluate people before they ever receive the medicine, and if it looks like they have psychological problems or physical problems, there's a long list of exclusion criteria. By the time a person has cleared all those and is ready to have the trial, you can be reasonably confident that they can handle it, that there are no psychological problems that can't be dealt with, that they don't have preexisting psychosis, and that they're physically able to handle it. That's the value of clinical studies. They don't just go into it half-cocked if you will.

Unregulated Mind-Body Medicine Abroad

DM: One of the aspects of ayahuasca that perhaps other psychedelics like psilocybin, for example, don't bring is very much a sense that it is mind-body medicine. It certainly works on the mind, but it also works on the body, and some of the research with the UDV supports this—you know, it's good for you. Not only is it good for your head, but it's good for your immune system, for example.

RLM: Would you say the same thing about LSD?

DM: The work hasn't been done, but it's less so. LSD is more cerebral. Ayahuasca gets in there and fixes your body. There is an I-thou relationship set up in the experience. You definitely have a feeling that it is fixing physical problems. In some of the more radical episodes that people have described, the spirit doctors come and open up your chest and take out your heart and work on it and put it back in.*

RLM: God, you make it sound so good. I wish I could go to Safeway and buy a bunch and just take some tonight.

DN: Well, but then it wouldn't work! You have to have the shaman and the context.

RLM: The set and the setting.

DM: Ideally, people go to South America and find these healing centers, and they have the experience. That's probably a good model. The problem with that is now ayahuasca tourism is quite popular, and so they're not all on the up and up. I mean sometimes the ayahuasca is not good quality. You kind of have to know the ropes down there to know who the good shamans are and which ones are charlatans.

RLM: There's no FDA for ayahuasca down there?

DM: There's no FDA regulation of ayahuasca in South America, although there are discussions in Peru that there should be

---

*McKenna notes, "Since I gave this interview in 2011 I had that experience once and it was quite transformative."

something like a union or a council of ayahuasqueros. If you're a member of the union then you're in good standing.*

RLM: Sure, or maybe eventually there will be consumer reports.

DM: Something like this. There is a need for quality control because now it's getting so popular that everybody is jumping on board. The real ayahuasqueros—because it's not something that you get into casually—have to know what they're doing, and there's quite a lot of training that goes into it.

RLM: I just want to underline something you said that's also in Jim Fadiman's latest book, *The Psychedelic Explorer's Guide,* and that's the importance of set and setting—preparing the day before to take the medicine with the proper person and then having time to process it the next day. Isn't that important for what you're talking about?

DM: Those are the key things to keep in mind.

•••

Cheerleader for Psychedelic Research

As we know from chapter 2, Rick Doblin is by far the world's foremost cheerleader for psychedelic research. As I mentioned before, I met him in 1985 at Esalen, where he was full of enthusiasm for his dream. He planned on going to Harvard, getting a PhD, and then founding a pharmaceutical company that would fund research around the world into psychedelics. He accomplished all of these things and more. His insights into ayahuasca in the following interview are invaluable.

---

*"The Ayahuasca Dialogues Report: Preliminary Research and Prospects for Safer and More Sustainable Ayahuasca," with a foreword by Dennis McKenna, Ethnobotanical Stewardship Council (ESC), November 2014, www.ethnobotanicalcouncil.org/wp-content/uploads/2014/11/ESC_AyaDialogues-Report_Nov2014_engl.pdf (accessed April 30, 2017).

The Science of the Sacred
Rick Doblin, PhD
March 2, 2013

RICK DOBLIN, PHD, is the founder and executive director of the Multidisciplinary Association for Psychedelic Studies (MAPS). He received his doctorate in public policy from Harvard's Kennedy School of Government, where he wrote his dissertation on the regulation of the medical uses of psychedelics and marijuana. His professional goal is to help develop legal contexts for the beneficial uses of psychedelics and marijuana, primarily as prescription medicines but also for personal growth for otherwise healthy people, and eventually to become a legally licensed psychedelic therapist.

From the Amazon to the Laboratory
Standardizing Ayahuasca for Scientific Analysis

RLM: Let's talk about ayahuasca. Jordi Riba has been conducting some research in Spain.

Rick Doblin, PhD (RD): Yes, Jordi is in Barcelona, and for the past fifteen years he has been able to work with ayahuasca. In its normal state, ayahuasca is a tea made of two different plants. In a research setting the dose has to be standardized so that it's reliable and repeatable, so that you can understand the results and compare them to each other. Jordi Riba and his team in Spain have a large batch of ayahuasca. They freeze dry it and encapsulate it in powder form. It's standardized and stays stable, so in that form it can be used in clinical research. Jordi has concentrated on what are called Phase I studies, which try to assess the safety, the mechanism of action, and basically how these drugs work—the metabolism of the drug, not therapeutic applications. He's creating a basis of scientific information about the safety and about possible uses that will facilitate future research with ayahuasca in therapeutic uses.

We worked with a team on a study where a Peruvian shaman came up to British Columbia and worked with First Nations people who have a high incidence of alcoholism and drug abuse. The Canadian psychiatrist Gabor Maté, MD, facilitated the process. They focused on the treatment of addiction, and they have gotten some remarkable results that are just being published.

Unfortunately, because ayahuasca contains DMT, a Schedule I drug, Health Canada sent a message to Gabor Maté saying that if he were to continue this work they would take away his medical license, and it would be considered a crime. But they also said that they would be open to trying to facilitate research through Health Canada.*

We actually had a donor interested in making some of this freeze-dried encapsulated ayahuasca and then trying to work through the Health Canada regulatory system to get it accepted for use, but the Peruvian shaman refused to do the work. They said that ayahuasca comes in a traditional format—this tea—and they didn't want it manipulated in this scientific way in a Western therapeutic context.

What's Driving the Popularity of Ayahuasca?

RLM: Why is there so much interest in ayahuasca both nationally in our country as well as in Europe now? One hears that it is attracting a great amount of attention.

RD: It is, and there's a couple of different reasons for it. One of the main reasons is that the use of ayahuasca began in a religious context. Much of the use in the United States has been spread by two

---

*Michael Posner, "B.C. Doctor Agrees to Stop Using Amazonian Plant to Treat Addictions," GlobeandMail.com, November 2011, www.theglobeandmail.com/life /health-and-fitness/bc-doctor-agrees-to-stop-using-amazonian-plant-to-treat-addictions /article4250579/ (accessed April 30, 2017).

different churches—primarily the União do Vegetal [UDV] or the Union of the Plants and also by the Santo Daime. These two religions have defended a religious right to use it—particularly the UDV, which went all the way to the U.S. Supreme Court. Jeffrey Bronfman from the Canadian Bronfman family, who was the president of the UDV in the United States, spent about $3 million of his own money on legal fees and actually won a unanimous ruling in the Supreme Court, saying that his church had a religious right to use it—although the DEA still had to work out some ways to regulate it. So I think many people who would be reluctant to break the law to use LSD or MDMA would take ayahuasca.

There's a reasonable claim to be made that much of the use is religious and protected by religious freedom. So I think there's a way in which a lot of people are comfortable, you could say, in this gray area with ayahuasca.

RLM: But what are people looking for when they're taking ayahuasca— what's the goal?

RD: They're looking for deeply profound spiritual experiences and a sense of connection, a sense of energy, a sense of being in touch with their own unconscious and their own deeper levels of the mind.

One advantage of ayahuasca is that it's relatively short acting—a couple of hours. LSD or psilocybin is a six- to eight-hour experience. Sometimes people will take ayahuasca all night in a religious setting, but they're drinking cups of tea every couple hours. UDV ceremonies actually begin at 8 p.m. and end at midnight, at which point people are pretty well grounded again. But during that process it's very profound and intense. For a period of about an hour and a half there is this sense of light and energy—a sense of warmth. There's a lot of body energy. A lot of people do have nausea and vomiting. I mean, the ayahuasca tastes vile; it really tastes horrible. But there's that kind of physicality that is grounding, and so it's not as abstract of an experience as LSD.

RLM: The neuroethnobotanist Stephan Beyer, PhD, author of *Singing to the Plants* [Albuquerque: University of New Mexico Press, 2009], told me that ayahuasca was originally used as an emetic because the food and the water supplies down in the jungles were so compromised that they needed to find something that they could take to immediately get them to regurgitate, and that was one of the origins of the use of ayahuasca. It is very interesting that there is that emetic aspect.

Medicine or a Sacrament?

RLM: Do you see a future therapeutic and medicinal potential for this particular substance?

RD: Definitely. There's a fundamental question that we need to address first, and that is whether this is a sacred substance that should only be used in a religious context or this is a more neutral substance. Is this just a series of chemicals that has a religious framework put over it? Can it validly be used outside of a religious context, in a Western therapeutic context?

RLM: Great question for future research.

RD: I think it can, and I think the context makes an incredible amount of difference in the outcome of the experience. There's a certain kind of religious pride, you could say, or even religious egotism, where people will say, "You know, this substance is sacred, more than anything else." But if we want to look at it, everything is sacred.

RLM: That's right. Everything on the Earth is sacred.

RD: These tools—these substances—have a more powerful ability to generate spiritual experiences in the sense of connection and moving beyond our own ego. Things that people have repressed—that they haven't wanted to see about themselves or others—tend to come to the surface. You can look at the Western scientific endeavor and Enlightenment—the centuries-long tradition that has brought us this ability to understand the universe around us—as sacred as well. Therefore, I answer this question by saying, "Yes, these substances can be used in a variety of different contexts, including a desacralized, not religious but therapeutic context."

I think ayahuasca has tremendous potential because of the series of things it does in a relatively short period of time—bringing people to these profound states. With sufficient support, it can be channeled into a religious or a therapeutic setting. I think both are equally valid when approached with respect.

DMT
Ayahuasca's "Spirit Molecule"

RLM: The active ingredient in ayahuasca is N,N-dimethyltryptamine, or DMT. What can you tell us about Rick Strassman's research on dimethyltryptamine in New Mexico?*

RD: Well, Rick was the first person that was able to restart research with psychedelics, and he got permission in 1990. He approached it outside of a religious context, in a hospital setting—a scientific setting. He administered it intravenously, where it comes on faster. It's more disorienting. He found that people had a range of experiences. At the higher doses people were more frightened than they were enlightened.

The experience of DMT when taken intravenously is very short acting. The beauty of ayahuasca is that the DMT is deactivated in the gut, so it's not active orally, but when you mix it with an MAOI—a monoamine oxidase inhibitor—it inhibits the digestion of it in the gut

---

*Rick Strassman, *DMT: The Spirit Molecule: A Doctor's Revolutionary Research into the Biology of Near-Death and Mystical Experiences* (Rochester, VT: Park Street Press, 2000).

and makes it orally active. When it's orally active it has a longer onset. It lasts longer, and you can learn more from it. You have a period of time to get adjusted to it. You can stay in the space for forty-five minutes to an hour and a half, and then you can come down over the next hour or forty-five minutes to sort of integrate it.

By using intravenous administration—where it just hits you out of the blue, and you're in a really different state very quickly—it's not surprising that Rick Strassman talked a lot about people's fears and anxieties and that they had doses that were too high. He also talked a lot about people having the sense of energy spirits or that they were somehow in contact with these plants' energies—these spirits, or aliens. I think he went a bit far in his speculations that these were actually entities that existed independently of us somewhere and that the ayahuasca helped people to see them. Although I think it was a classic blindness. If you are a researcher giving people drugs intravenously in a hospital setting, and then subjects have these images of aliens experimenting on them, it's not that hard to suggest that maybe it's just symbolically what's actually going on with them in the hospital.

Know Before You Go
Risks of Ayahuasca Tourism

RLM: What are some of the dangers of ayahuasca?

RD: There have been a small number of people who have died. Some of the shamans have what you could call a poly-pharmacy. They will mix nicotine—tobacco—and other things in with the ayahuasca. Sometimes people have gotten nicotine poisoning and died.

RLM: Were the deaths you're aware of only in South America?

RD: Some were here in the United States, and some were in Canada. There is a recent tragic story of a young man who went down to Peru for an ayahuasca ceremony, where the model that they use is not so much a therapeutic or supportive model but more like a vision quest. They give people ayahuasca in a little hut in the jungle, and then they spend the next few days there. This young man died. The shaman tried to cover it up and buried him, but eventually it came out. These are remarkably rare circumstances.

We should also recognize that there are loads of people that are allergic to aspirin and die from it, and yet we consider it to be one of the safest drugs that we have. People are allergic to and die from penicillin. The dangers of ayahuasca are primarily psychological rather than physiological.

• • •

Present scientific research on ayahuasca is mostly anecdotal evidence gleaned over generations from shamans in South America. There is yet to be a series of scientifically controlled double-blind studies. Given that Jordi Riba in Barcelona has created a method of calibrating dosage* there will likely be new studies on the horizon, but it will be very slow growing. All scientists researching psychedelics report a minimum of funding for expensive research.

At the very same time people all over the world are using ayahuasca for healing and consciousness expansion in sub rosa gatherings, and the feedback continues to be overwhelmingly positive. While situations requiring medical intervention for ingestion of ayahuasca are rare, there is a measurable amount of risk involved with this substance. In distinction to LSD, psilocybin, and MDMA, there have been inconclusive deaths attributed to ayahuasca reported in South America. We are warned about the existence of South American tourist shamans who exploit their geography and local reputation by advertising ayahuasca seminars to the world.

Those considering joining an ayahuasca seminar are well advised

---

*Jordi Riba, and Manel J. Barbanoj, "A Pharmacological Study of Ayahuasca in Healthy Volunteers," *Bulletin of the Multidisciplinary Association for Psychedelic Studies* 8, no. 3 (Autumn 1998): 12–15.

to carefully research all medicines they are taking for potential negative interactions (some severe), to be prepared for a lengthy journey, and most of all to follow the proper procedures as described in this book.

Stunningly, some people have already trained themselves to move through daily life and do critical thinking under the effects of large doses of LSD by taking increasing doses over time. (The astrophysicist Carl Sagan and the founder of Apple are examples.) Only shamans function with volitional intention under the influence of ayahuasca.

FIVE

Psychiatric Prescription Drugs

Tired Soldiers

A Drug-Induced Epidemic of Disabling Mental Illness

Our society believes that psychiatric medications have led to a "revolutionary" advance in the treatment of mental disorders, and yet these pages tell of a drug-induced epidemic of disabling mental illness.

ROBERT WHITAKER, *ANATOMY OF AN EPIDEMIC:*
MAGIC BULLETS, PSYCHIATRIC DRUGS, AND THE
ASTONISHING RISE OF MENTAL ILLNESS IN AMERICA

I've been practicing psychology for almost fifty years, and this quote echoes what I have witnessed and observed during this period. Namely, that there is a drug-induced epidemic of disabling mental illness. This epidemic is not caused by illicit street drugs like cocaine, heroin, methamphetamine, and marijuana, but rather by prescription medicine given to patients all over the country.

This topic of pharmaceutical company–induced sickness is near and dear to my heart. When I took my first job as a psychologist back in 1961 at the Laconia State School for the Mentally Retarded and Emotionally Disturbed, I witnessed patients being wrapped in sail cloth from sailboats—heavy canvas—and sprayed with ice-cold water. Then they were rolled around on the ground and then sprayed again with ice-cold water. I witnessed patients being hit with what they called sock tranquilizers—where they would put pieces of soap in a woman's stocking and swing it and hit the patients. I witnessed electroconvulsive shock therapy given to patients in the cells that they lived in. It was shocking (pun intended). I was in my early twenties, and witnessing these physically abusive "treatments" was what I imagined a medieval torture chamber to look like. But I was not in a medieval torture chamber. I was in a hospital in New Hampshire and the year was 1961.

Today's interview may be the most important you have ever experienced if you or a family member or friend are suffering from some form of emotional, psychological, or intellectual challenges. If you're taking some form of psychoactive medicine, or if you are considering taking some form of psychoactive medicine, you will want to consider extremely carefully the following interview with award-winning journalist Robert Whitaker.

Whitaker was the director of publications at Harvard Medical School until 1994, when he cofounded the publishing company CenterWatch, which covered the pharmaceutical clinical-trials industry. He has spent a major part of his career investigating the pharmaceutical industry and their products.

Although the topic of his book, *Anatomy of an Epidemic,* is selective serotonin reuptake inhibitors, SSRIs, which are not technically considered psychedelics, they are psychoactive and thus have a profound influence on emotional and cognitive functioning. Whitaker's findings are so important that I felt compelled to include them.

Questioning the Psychiatric Paradigm
Robert Whitaker
December 6, 2011, and November 4, 2014

ROBERT WHITAKER is author of *Mad in America: Bad Science, Bad Medicine, and the Enduring Mistreatment of the Mentally Ill*. His book *Anatomy of an Epidemic: Magic Bullets, Psychiatric Drugs, and the Astonishing Rise of Mental Illness in America* won the 2010 Investigative Reporters and Editors Book Award for best investigative journalism. He has won numerous awards as a journalist covering medicine and science, including the George Polk Award for Medical Reporting and the National Association of Science Writers Award for best magazine article. In 1998, Robert cowrote a series on psychiatric research for the *Boston Globe* that was a finalist for the Pulitzer Prize for Public Service.

RLM: Robert, you wrote an article in the *Boston Globe* in 1998 about the mentally ill being given chemical agents that heightened their psychosis, is that correct?

Robert Whitaker (RW): That's true.

RLM: Talk a bit about your *Boston Globe* series and how schizophrenia has worsened over twenty years, and then please tell us about how poor countries are having better outcomes with schizophrenia than the richer ones.

RW: Initially, in that series, we were writing about abuses of patients in psychiatric research settings. One of the abuses we wrote about were studies in which people came into emergency rooms experiencing psychotic symptoms, and the psychiatrists, rather than treat them in a way designed to help diminish those symptoms and agitation, instead gave them agents that they expected would make them worse—amphetamines and ketamine, that sort of thing. The idea was that if they gave them different agents expected to make them worse, this would lead to some understanding of the possible chemical problems that were going on with the person at the time of their psychosis.

Imagine you're suffering, or you're struggling with your mind. Or maybe it's one of your brothers or sisters or your son or daughter, and you take them to an emergency room where you expect they are to be helped, and instead they are put in an experiment where they are given chemical agents designed to heighten their symptoms. The informed consent forms for those experiments misleadingly stated that they were being given an experimental drug that may or may not help, but that was not so at all. You wouldn't do this to people coming in suffering from heart pains. You wouldn't give them some agent to make their pain worse. So that was my introduction into this very odd world of how we treat those said to be mentally ill.

In the *Globe* series, we also wrote about studies in which researchers had withdrawn antipsychotic medications from patients diagnosed with schizophrenia. At that time, I had a completely conventional understanding of psychiatric drugs. I thought that antipsychotic drugs fixed a chemical imbalance in the brain and acted like insulin for diabetes. I thought they were absolutely essential. So I asked myself, "Why would you ever run studies in which you had withdrawn a drug that was seen as so essential?" Later, as we'll see, I came to rethink this understanding based on some information I began to uncover while doing the research for that *Boston Globe* series.

The Schizophrenia Conundrum
Better Results with Fewer Meds

RLM: What happened with that *Boston Globe* series?

RW: Well, first of all, I came upon two studies done by the World Health Organization that compared outcomes in three poor countries—specifically India, Nigeria, and Colombia—with longer-term outcomes in the United States and five other "developed countries." Each time, they found that the outcomes were much better in the poor countries—specifically India and Nigeria. They even concluded that living in a developed country—a rich country like the United States—is "a strong predictor" that if you're diagnosed with schizophrenia, you won't have a good outcome.

So I'm wondering, "Why would that be?" I looked further into the studies, and after the first such study, the researchers hypothesized that maybe the reason for the better outcomes in the poor countries was that they were more medication compliant—they took their antipsychotics more regularly. That makes sense as a hypothesis, if you believe the drugs are so essential. They measured medication usage in the second study and found, much to their surprise, that the opposite was true. In the poor countries, they used the drugs acutely, for a short period of time, but they did not keep their patients on the drugs long-term. In the poor countries, only 16 percent of schizophrenia patients were continually maintained on antipsychotics, whereas in the United States and other developed countries, that was the standard of care for all patients.

All of a sudden I was presented with this finding that went against what I had just written for the *Boston Globe,* which was that the drugs were essential. Yet here in this cross-cultural study, you found better outcomes where they were using the drugs much more sparingly.

The second thing was that when I was doing that series with the *Boston Globe,* I had a completely conventional understanding of psychiatry's history. I believed that we were coming to understand that the biology of major mental disorders like schizophrenia was caused by chemical imbalances and that we had drugs to fix those chemical imbalances. We had a new generation of antipsychotics, which were better than the first generation. That's a story of medical progress.

Then I came upon a study by Harvard researchers that looked at longer-term outcomes over the past century, and they came up with two conclusions. First, modern outcomes today were no better than they had been in the first third of the twentieth century, long before the drugs came on the market. And second, outcomes had actually *worsened* in the previous fifteen years. So again, this belied the story of progress that I thought to be true. It was those studies that made me curious and made me want to investigate further about treatments for the mentally ill—those labeled mad, schizophrenic, and so forth—and why we are getting such bad outcomes today. That is what led me on this long journalistic enterprise.

The Early History of Psychiatric Treatment

1751: Patients Treated as Animals in the "Age of Reason"

RLM: So here we have an investigative reporter who discovers that people going into emergency rooms are being given chemical agents that heighten their psychosis and mental illness rather than reduce it. He finds out that outcome studies for schizophrenia in the United States indicate that results are worse over the past fifteen years than they were in the early part of the century. And furthermore, he finds out that countries like India and Nigeria have had better outcomes than countries like the United States while prescribing fewer drugs.

Take us back to 1751, when Benjamin Franklin petitions the assembly in Pennsylvania for a mental hospital. What kind of attitudes did people have back then about people suffering from mental illness? We're going to look at the history of this and how it informs how we're treating the mentally ill today.

RW: Once I began investigating this, it became clear to me that we need to use history to understand how we treat and think about the mentally ill today. So I decided to trace the treatment of the seriously mentally ill in the book *Mad in America,* from colonial times until today. While Pennsylvania was still a colony of England, Benjamin Franklin and others opened the first hospital in the colonies. They said they would have a section that would take care of the mad. In the basement of the hospital, they basically built a number of cells and furnished them with straw as if they were stalls for animals. Once they opened the hospital, the mad would be put in those basement cells. There was a window just a little bit above the ground, and during the weekend or on Sunday, people from Philadelphia could come in and actually pay a few cents to look at the crazy people in the cells, almost as if they were going to a zoo.

RLM: Now what's going on at this time?

RW: In medical textbooks, the thought at this time—the "age of reason"—was that the mad, by virtue of having lost their reason, have descended to a lower level of being and are a sort of animal. So the way to treat the mad is to instill fear in them and treat them harshly. They thought the mad were insensitive to heat and cold and didn't need clothes in those cells. Documents from the hospital talk about how the person who oversaw the mad was like a keeper of the animals—he had whips and shackles and that sort of thing. So at this very early moment in the treatment of the seriously mentally ill, we have a conception of them as less than human—as having descended to a lower level of being and that they needed to be treated harshly in order to be kept in line.

RLM: They were called brutes, weren't they?

RW: Absolutely, and that's a reflection of how they were conceived.

RLM: Didn't Benjamin Rush put some kind of paste on them to make their skin blister?

RW: Yes, absolutely. Benjamin Rush is remembered today as the father of American psychiatry. He brought back the teachings from Europe, and the idea was that you needed to use medical therapies that in some ways weakened the patient.

If you could give them something to make them vomit over and over again or make them have diarrhea over and over again, you would deplete them and make them weaker. In that weakened state they would no longer be able to be so agitated, or so difficult, or so angry with their keepers.

So you see in the medical texts that Rush adopted in the 1700s, there were a number of therapies that were in fact designed to weaken them—in fact make them sick or make them dizzy. To do that, they would spin them around and around and around.

RLM: Benjamin Rush invented a chair—I read in your book—to make them spin and make them weak.

RW: There were actually two different things. There was a spinning device that Rush used—but that one was actually invented in Europe. You would just put people on a spinning disk and run them around until they would throw up, and then they would crawl back to their cells and wouldn't bother anybody for a while. Rush invented something called the tranquilizer chair. He believed that madness was due to a blood imbalance and that madness was caused by too much blood rushing to the head. So he bled his people profusely. They would be bound into this chair, kept there from anywhere from four hours to several days, and be bled while having ice dumped on their head, all of which drained blood from the overheated brain.

Now imagine that you're wrapped in this chair for three or four days, with ice being poured on your head. You're going to be pretty weak at the end of that time, and you're going to be quieter, because you're going to be so exhausted; and that's what Rush talks about—he says after a certain length of time people become composed, quieter, and more tranquil. He talked about how satisfied he was. This chair, which you can still see in some museums, was then exported to Europe and it became the first psychiatric medical therapy, so to speak, developed in the United States and then exported to Europe.

RLM: So you strap a person in a chair, you pour ice water on their head, you spin them in the chair, you purge them, and you take blood out of their system. You force them to vomit and you blister their skin, and then you say, "Lo and behold—this is a nice, docile person we have here."

RW: Exactly, and if we did a clinical trial of Rush's chair today, we'd probably see, as an effect, a more manageable person who would be expressing fewer psychotic symptoms. We laugh about these therapies from long ago, but if the goal is to make people more manageable and quieter, those early therapies indeed did that.

RLM: Very unfortunate, because Benjamin Rush, who was also one of the signers of the Declaration of Independence and the foremost physician in the United States, went from being a Quaker humanitarian to using these almost barbaric techniques. I know he ruined his reputation eventually in the United States because he purged too many people of blood and too many of them died from it.

1812: The Temporary Sanity of "Moral Treatment"

RLM: Take us forward now to about 1812, to the beginning of what's called "moral treatment."

RW: We forget this part of history. In conventional histories of psychiatry there is a sense that the mentally ill were always mistreated in the past, but if you really look in the history you find this era when "moral therapy" held sway. It was a reform movement that came out of York, England, ushered in by Quakers there, who looked at how one of their own people had been mistreated in mental hospitals in England and said, "We don't know what causes madness, but we do know they are brethren. As brethren we're going to develop a form of care that treats them as fellow human beings." There is this reconception—they are not animals. The York Quakers built a retreat out in the countryside because they thought that nature could be healing. There, the people were treated as ordinarily as possible. They were dressed in normal clothes. They had ordinary bedrooms. They would have entertainment in the evening. There were walks in the country and gardening, because they thought that exercise was good. The Quakers would feed them four meals a day, and they believed in a little bit of sherry in the afternoon. So what happened?

The Quakers found a couple things: the resistance of patients and the propensity for violence pretty much disappears, because they're not being treated so aggressively. They found that many people with this kind treatment got well after just twelve months.

RW: After some time in the country, many people never needed to come back to the asylum. After the Quakers in York, England, pioneered this in the very last years of the 1700s, it gets imported into the United States by Quakers here, and we started getting these moral therapy asylums dotting major East Coast cities.

There was one in Philadelphia, one in Boston, and one in Hartford. Researchers today have gone back and looked at their records and have concluded that there has probably never been a more effective form of care in the United States.

They found that more than 50 percent of the newly admitted would be discharged within twelve months. The best long-term study we have, which went for about thirty years, found that something like 50 percent of first-episode patients, who were then discharged, never returned to the asylum.

RLM: And these were places that were called asylums—they were actually small homelike facilities, weren't they?

RW: Yes, exactly. I mean, we're using the word "asylum" in the old sense of the word—as a refuge, not as a mental hospital but a time-out place from the rigors of daily life. They were meant to be comfortable, small, and architecturally pleasing. People wanted pleasing grounds where they could walk and such. So in terms of a humanistic ethical form of care, we can look back to these early retreats from

1812 to 1850, more or less, and rediscover a form of care that would be great if we could duplicate it today.

1859: From Darwinian Evolution to Galtonian Eugenics

RLM: So after this "moral treatment," what came next?

RW: The next big swing in our conceptions of the mentally ill happens post-Darwin. Darwin writes his *Origin of Species* in the mid-1800s, and although he doesn't really talk about humans, it's obvious that humans evolved. Then his cousin Sir Francis Galton picks up on this. He says that if a human society wants to prosper, it needs to take those with good germ plasm and encourage them to breed and have kids as well as identify those with bad germ plasm to prevent them from breeding.

Galton is from England, but it's in the United States that leaders really embrace this idea. So the eugenics policy that then gets enacted into law first happens in the United States before anywhere else. Once you accept this idea—in order to prosper, a society has to prevent those with bad germ plasm from breeding—you can see what society needs to do. It needs to begin distinguishing between people it calls *fit* and those it deems *unfit*.

As America adopts eugenic attitudes, democracy becomes a ridiculous idea because not all men are in fact created equal. Now once you start trying to identify the unfit, who comes at the top of that list? Of course, it's the mentally ill.

1896: Imprisonment and Sterilization

RW: Beginning in 1896, eugenicists in the United States began passing policies designed to prevent "the mad" from breeding. First, they pass laws saying it's illegal for the insane to marry. Next, they start locking people up and keeping them in hospitals for long periods of time—at least until they pass their breeding years. Once these ideas really take hold—around 1900—people stop being discharged from the mental hospitals, and we had huge growth in the number of institutionalized people. Once you were declared insane or mentally ill, it became very hard to get out.

RLM: Definitely. Remember when I said earlier in the program that my first job was at a mental hospital in 1961? I remember distinctly interviewing a man there who just talked to me as a peer, and I said to him, "I can tell that you're just talking to me 'regular.' Why are you here?" He said, "Because they'll never let me out."

RW: Yeah. You see this in the records—it's just tragic. People coming in when they're eighteen to twenty-five who often had a lot of difficulties that preceded their time in the hospital and then they never get out.

RLM: Yes, I also met people, at the time, who were in the hospital for twenty or twenty-five years because their families wanted to get rid of them.

RW: You have that as well, of course. Then we began sterilizing the mentally ill too, and that was deemed constitutional by the U.S. Supreme Court in 1927.

RLM: We were the first country that had sterilization. In fact, I think I read in your book that 80 percent of the sterilizations in the United States happened right here in California where I'm broadcasting from.

RW: I don't remember the percentage, but California was certainly a leader in this whole initiative, so much so that when Hitler wanted to start a sterilization program in Germany he actually sent some of his scientists to California.

RLM: Wow.

1918: Insanity as Genetically Determined

RLM: Moving into the twentieth century, this germ-plasm theory is the foundation for our current notion of schizophrenia. We're thinking it's something in the genes—that is passed on from generation to generation—that must be stopped in some way.

RW: The eugenicists wanted to say that people were genetically determined. The whole point was to identify people with bad germ plasm. The science of eugenics was really promoted with the pursuit of scholarly activity at some of the best universities in United States—I mean, Ivy League universities. This wasn't some sort of fringe endeavor—this was done at the heart of American academics. By around 1918, there were texts that said insanity is a single-gene recessive disorder, like blue eyes. So if you get the normalcy gene from say, your father, and the insane gene from your mother, you will be a carrier but you will be normal. But if you get an insane gene from father and an insane gene from mother, then you're going to be insane.

RLM: So they're saying that insanity is a recessive gene.

RW: Yes. There was never any good science behind this, but state and county fairs in the 1920s had exhibits by the American Eugenics Society that said: "Every eight minutes another insane person is born." They would call this a burden on society. Around this time we begin to see the stigmatization of the mentally ill in history, as they were being seen or conceived of as a real burden on society. We were spending a lot of money on these people. Now and then you would see a book asking whether we should just be killing these people instead of housing them.

1930s: Coma and Convulsive Therapies—
Old Methodology, New Technology

RLM: So, we're going from 1751, where the mentally ill are considered animals in cells lying on straw, to the twentieth century, where people are talking about doing away with them—there's sterilization going on—and then along comes World War II, which brings us into hydrotherapy, shock therapy, and convulsive therapy.

RW: In the 1930s you see the number of therapies increase dramatically. You have something called insulin coma therapy, where you'd give someone a shot of insulin—so much that they would go into shock—and then you'd administer sugar to bring them back. You would do this repetitively. But it just made people quieter. They became childlike because they felt grateful to the therapist for reviving them. With insulin coma therapy, you could actually see repetitive signs of brain damage in an autopsy. But again, it made people more manageable and childlike.

We also got something called metrazol convulsive therapy. Metrazol was a poison that caused convulsions so severe that people would break their teeth or possibly fracture bones in their back. As that is introduced, you also see people changing after you had this poison administered. But people were so afraid of it in the asylums, you could just threaten them with metrazol convulsive therapy and they would often get in line and become quieter.

After this we get electroshock therapy. Electroshock is initially ushered into mental hospitals for the same reason that metrazol convulsive therapy was. The idea was that these seizures were good for people, and electricity became an easier way to induce these seizures. But again, the initial reports were all about how it makes them quieter—they don't even remember who they are after they come out, and they're more childlike.

RLM: We know Ernest Hemingway received a series of electroshock therapies prior to his suicide.

RW: That's the thing—to the public this therapy is being presented as a miracle cure, but in the case studies it was recognized that these were brain-damaging therapies. Some theorists posited that perhaps some people, that is, the mad, do better with less brain function, and of course, ultimately, this leads to prefrontal lobotomy.

1940: The Prefrontal Lobotomy

RW: A Portuguese neurologist, Edgar Moniz, claimed that if you destroy the frontal lobe, people are quieted and the madness goes away. This gets imported into the United States, and in 1940 it is treated as a miracle.

RLM: The prefrontal lobotomy was considered a miracle?

RW: Yeah. Walter Freeman was the big promoter of it in the United States. He would go around from hospital to hospital and destroy thirty to forty people's frontal lobes in one day. There was even talk that maybe the frontal lobes are like the appendix and that we don't really need them.

RLM: We go from almost waterboarding to spinning, to puking, to purging, taking out the blood, to wet wraps, on to insulin shock, and then electroshock, and now finally Dr. Freeman comes up with the ultimate way to make the mentally ill docile, which is to cut out a major piece of their brain.

RW: Right, and it's not just any piece of the brain. It's the prefrontal lobes. This is the part that makes us human. If you look at a chimpanzee brain and a human brain, the difference is that you see in the human brain the pronounced frontal lobes. This is the part of the brain thought to be the seat of consciousness. This is the part that worries about the future and monitors our actions. The mentally ill were somehow seen as not in need of this part of their brain. But again, while the press was treating it as a miracle brain surgery—Edgar Moniz even wins the Nobel Prize in Medicine for inventing it—you then read the actual case descriptions. They talk about people no longer caring about the world or themselves.

Modern Drugs for Modern Times
Antipsychotics, Benzodiazepines, and SSRIs

1955: Antipsychotics—Lobotomy in a Pill

RLM: Take us from lobotomies to the modern era, beginning with Thorazine [chlorpromazine], the first antipsychotic.

RW: Thorazine arrived in mental hospitals in 1954, kicking off what is remembered today as a great psychopharmacological revolution—a "Great Leap Forward" in care. Remember, they're called antipsychotics today, as if they're antidotes to psychosis; but, when they were first introduced, they were actually lauded as causing a change in being similar to that of a surgical lobotomy. The people touting the drugs even say, "It's as if the drug causes a chemical lobotomy." But that is not seen as a bad thing in 1954; that's seen as a good thing, because Edgar Moniz had just won the Nobel Prize in Medicine for his discovery of the therapeutic value of lobotomy. This change from an agitated person—someone with wild thoughts—into a quieter person—someone who shuffles along and doesn't care, who's disinterested in the world—was seen as a good thing. Well, it might be a good thing for the people managing the asylum, but is it a good thing for the person himself or herself?

This is so important. Our common understanding is that drugs represent a break from these problems of the past. Yet you go back to the 1950s and they're seen as a continuation of what we've been doing rather than a break. It's important to note that early on they're seen as "tranquilizers," called neuroleptics [taking hold of the nerves], but then they get reconceptualized in the public mind as "antipsychotics," as if they're antibiotics. They're seen as an antidote to psychosis.

Moving forward, we see a new story emerge—that all of these drugs fix chemical imbalances in the brain like insulin does with diabetes. And if that metaphor is true, that is a story of great advance. It means you've identified the pathology of a disorder and now you have a treatment that is specific to it.

But now you look into the science, and once again you find that's not true. You find that we still don't know the pathology of depression or of psychosis. They never found that people with a certain diagnosis had a characteristic chemical imbalance. Also, you find that you can't say that the drugs correct a chemical imbalance. Moreover, you see a subjective value in the ratings of these drugs. If someone is quieter, moves around less, and is less aggressive, then this is seen as evidence that the drug works in a medical way. But we could take the old view and say that these antipsychotics are causing a change in being that makes them more acceptable to others.

RLM: Yes—they're becoming zombielike. We can't get away from your original findings, which showed developed countries are doing worse than people from undeveloped countries who take fewer of the medicines, in countries such as Nigeria and India.

RW: In the aggregate, that's absolutely true. In terms of doing worse, there are several elements of this. People on medication long-term actually are more likely to still be psychotic at ten and fifteen years later, whereas, on the whole, those who go off the medications see a diminishment of psychotic symptoms starting around year two, such that over the long-term they are much less likely to still be psychotic. That is what we see in a long-term study by Martin Harrow.

People in these poorer countries, once off the medication long-term, are much more likely to be employed. They're much more likely to be in school. They're much more likely to have some sort of decent social life, and they are, frankly, much, much less likely to be psychotic long-term than those who stay on antipsychotics continuously. What you see in those who stay on antipsychotics continuously—and there's a minority who do well on them—the majority live quiet lives of desperation or often end up physically ill and unemployed . . . not the sort of life anyone would wish for their son or daughter.

RLM: Mental illness is on a continuum, and the schizophrenics are at the edge of the continuum. Let's talk about the regular people; in this country, millions are suffering from depression and anxiety and are taking various forms of these psychoactive medications. Give us a little history about how benzodiazepines came about.

RW: Benzodiazepines grew out of post–World War II research where people were looking for a magic bullet for Gram-negative bacteria. Penicillin works on what's called Gram-positive bacteria, a different type of bacteria, and researchers were looking for a magic bullet for this other type of bacteria. They found that one of the chemicals they came up with in initial animal testing had an odd effect—it basically caused muscle paralysis in rats, which was reversible. The researchers noted the rats were not distressed by this sudden paralysis. The researchers said, "Aha, this agent has a tranquilizing effect. It blocks the ability of the body to mount an emotional response." This line of research eventually leads to the first benzodiazepines—drugs like Librium [chlordiazepoxide] and Valium [diazepam].

They were brought to market in the early '60s [we hear about "Mother's Little Helper" and that sort of thing] as nonaddictive drugs. But it becomes clear pretty fast that while they're very effective in knocking down anxiety over the short term, that effect begins to wear off after four to six weeks; and then, when people try to come off, they have extreme withdrawal symptoms and get what's called rebound anxiety, where they are now worse than they were when they went on the pill. Because of that, by the end of the 1970s the governments of the United States and the United Kingdom both said, "Wow! These drugs are addictive. We need to limit them to short-term use." In fact, it was Betty Ford's physician who said in the late '70s that benzodiazepines were one of the biggest drug problems we had in this country at that time.

RLM: The First Lady was on Valium?

RW: Yes, but what's so remarkable is that you still see physicians prescribing benzodiazepines in spite of this understanding of the drugs—that while they are very effective for about a week or two weeks, they lose that effectiveness and then you're into this situation where you can have a problematic withdrawal period when you come off. If you stay on, the research is quite clear that you get physical and emotional decline, increased anxiety, and often agoraphobia—where people can't go out of the house. You see increasing disability. All of that's really solid in the research literature.

In modern times, they're becoming part of a usual drug cocktail, which is really astonishing because no one is even claiming that benzodiazepines are good for you long term and yet that's how they're being used—incorporated into prescribing patterns.

RLM: Yes. It's very important that we tell our listeners the actual names of the medicines that are in this family of benzodiazepines. Of course, the older generation was Miltown [meprobamate], and then we had Librium. Remember the old slogan, "Give me Librium or give me meth?" We now have Ativan [lorazepam] and Xanax [alprazolam]—which is very popular all over the United States—and we have Klonopin [clonazepam]. What have I missed?

RW: Those are the big three right now. The market for benzodiazepines was declining in the 1970s with the understanding that Librium and Valium could be so addictive. And sure enough, Xanax was then promoted as a nonaddictive drug when it was brought to market. But when you look at the research in which they tested Xanax, you found that it was very effective for about four weeks. By the end of six weeks, it was not really much more effective than placebo. Then they did a withdrawal study, and by the end of that withdrawal study, the Xanax patients were so much worse than the placebo patients. You see rebound anxiety and you see all sorts of other adverse effects.

But unfortunately, the people being paid by the makers of Xanax to do that trial—academic psychiatrists at academic medical centers—didn't focus on the withdrawal problem. They didn't focus on how rebound anxiety got so much worse. They didn't even focus on the six-week results. When they published their results, they focused on this shorter, four-week period of time when Xanax is supposedly very effective. There was even talk about how it was nonaddictive. It's just nonsense. I get emails every day from people who are in despair—locked into a benzodiazepine addiction, just can't get off—and it has ruined their lives.

1980s: SSRIs and the Epidemic of Mental Illness

RLM: Let's now talk about your research into the selective serotonin reuptake inhibitors, SSRIs.

RW: Part of the conventional narrative of progress is that in 1987, Prozac [fluoxetine] arrives on the market. This is the first SSRI and the first of the *second-generation* psychiatric drugs—this next step up this ladder of progress. Generally in medicine, when you see progress—when you see new therapies arrive—the burden that disorder takes in terms of disability and so forth *lessens* in society. It makes sense that the burden that disorder takes on your society should, at the very least, stay the same or improve since you have an effective new treatment for a disorder.

RLM: For example, Jonas Salk comes up with a vaccine, and polio is decreased.

RW: Exactly. Instead, our disability rates due to mental disorders have steadily risen during this era of the psychopharmacological revolution—the number of people unable to function well in society and in need of government care. In absolute numbers, it's basically risen from around 360,000 adults in 1955 to more than 4.7 million adults today. In the past twenty years we've really embraced this paradigm of care, and what has happened to disability rates? In 1987,

1.25 million adults were on disability, receiving a government payment because of mental illness. Today, there are around 4.7 million people receiving such payments. During this time of increased use of second-generation psychiatric drugs, we have had a fourfold increase in the number of adults on disability.

And, of course, we're now medicating kids. We didn't used to do that. In 1987, there were 16,200 children whose families received a disability payment because they were "severely mentally ill." Today we're well over 600,000 kids—so during the past twenty-five years we've had a thirty-five-fold increase in severely disabled children due to mental disorders. If you follow those kids who go on disability as children, when they hit age eighteen, about two-thirds are going right onto adult disability, and they basically now have a life as a mental patient laid out before them. Those numbers do not tell of a form of care that is lessening the burden of psychiatric distress in our society. Instead they tell us exactly the opposite.

RLM: Is there any substantial evidence that people who are depressed have different brain chemistry than the rest of us?

RW: The idea is that people who are depressed have low amounts of the neurotransmitter serotonin. This arose not from investigations into people who are depressed but by understanding how drugs and antidepressants acted on the brain. Just to simplify this: Prozac and the other SSRIs block the reuptake of serotonin from the synaptic cleft between neurons, therefore theoretically increasing serotonergic activity. People have hypothesized that maybe depression is due to low serotonin, but they found that prior to going on medication, depressed people had nothing abnormal with their serotonergic system. The psychiatric community failed to communicate that finding, which goes back to the early 1980s, to the American public. Is there evidence that people with depression suffer from an abnormal serotonergic system? Not before they go on the drug. After the drug, we see that may be the case.

RLM: To visualize the synaptic clefts that Bob is talking about, picture some wiring in your house running along the baseboard, and every once in a while there's a little junction box, and from the junction box wires go out to various other areas of the house. We're made the same way—we've got electrical wiring, and it goes into these little boxes where all this neurochemistry takes place, and then it goes out to other places. When we close the exit doors in the junction box, the neurotransmitting chemicals, which are inside the box, are trapped and thus they increase in concentration. That's what a reuptake inhibitor does. It closes off some little doors in that box, so the chemicals can't go out, and the chemicals build up inside the box.

Long-Term Consequences of Antidepressants
How the Brain Maintains Homeostasis

RLM: The medical profession decided it was their genetics that made psychiatric patients "different" from the rest of us. Bob is telling us that those who are depressed do not have a different brain chemistry. An important question thus arises, what happens if you take people who have the same brain chemistry as the rest of us and then give them something to change their brain chemistry?

RW: The irony is that once we understood how drugs act on the brain, researchers hypothesized that depression was due to low serotonergic activity. So now you go on an SSRI, which upsurges serotonergic activity in the brain. The brain, being this extraordinarily neuroplastic organ, now tries to compensate for the presence of that drug. So what does it do? Since the drug is upping serotonergic activity, the brain actually down-regulates or decreases its own serotonergic activity. So the neuron—that wire that's coming up to the gap [synapse]—starts releasing less serotonin than normal. And then the receiving postsynaptic neuron actually decreases the density of its receptors for serotonin. You can see why this is:

researchers say the brain is trying to maintain homeostatic equilibrium, its normal functioning. They found that prior to going on an antidepressant, you don't have this problem. But once you are on the drug for a longer period of time, you do. So the drug actually induces the very abnormality hypothesized to cause depression in the first place.

Antidepressants may be the most commonly prescribed drugs in America. In terms of their short-term efficacy, they beat placebo, but only for those with severe symptoms. That's where you see a clear benefit over placebo in the short term—in the severely ill—but not for those with mild or moderate depression. But when you start looking at long-term outcomes, you find time and time again that while medicated people may initially get better a little quicker, they seem to relapse back into depression more frequently than before they were using antidepressants. As early as the 1970s you see some psychiatrists saying, "I think these drugs are causing a chronification of the disease. People aren't staying well as long as they used to after recovering from an episode."

2012: The Exercise Study

RLM: Correct me if I'm off here, but I thought the Duke University study comparing an SSRI with exercise indicated that the SSRI actually made people worse.

RW: The Duke study is quite clear. There were three groups: One, drug; two, drug plus exercise; and three, exercise alone. The hypothesis was that the drug plus exercise would do the best at the end of ten months. At the end of about sixteen weeks, the drug-treated patients were doing a little bit better than the exercise-alone group. But then between sixteen weeks and roughly forty-four weeks, the exercise-alone patients continued to get better, whereas those on the drug alone or drug plus exercise had many relapses. Only 30 percent of the exercise-alone group was still depressed at the end of ten months, whereas around 55 percent of the drug-plus-exercise group were now depressed. In that study, the drugs can be seen as acting as an anchor, weighing down or subtracting from the exercise group, rather than being an added benefit.

RLM: And Duke University replicated that study about four or five years after the original one and found the same thing.

RW: That's pretty compelling, but there are a number of studies like this. One of the underappreciated studies was called the STAR*D study—the largest antidepressant trial ever conducted—of 4,041 patients. This trial was funded by the National Institute of Mental Health [NIMH] and was supposed to guide future care. Here were the bottom-line results: Of the 4,041 patients at the end of one year, there were only 108 patients who remitted* and then never relapsed and stayed in the trial for the year. All the others never remitted, relapsed, or dropped out of the trial. So that's a documented stay-well rate of 3 percent, which is the worst outcome I've ever seen in a longer-term antidepressant study.

RLM: This is right from the National Institutes of Health website: "The most common side effects associated with SSRIs include headache, nausea, sleeplessness or drowsiness, agitation, sexual problems . . ." and they go on to say they're popular because they do not cause many side effects. So, I take this drug because I'm depressed, and then I get sexual problems. I get anxiety. I can't sleep well. I've got a headache, but I'm reading here "not many side effects," and I start to think, what's going on with me? Am I different from everybody else? Getting these negative effects and thinking I should not be getting negative effects almost assuredly will make me feel much worse.

---

*Patients experienced lessening of symptoms.

Following the Money
Bad Incentives in Psychiatry and the Rise of Big Pharma

RLM: Let's follow the money—what's going on here from a monetary point of view?

RW: You can see that it is a commercial enterprise. We were spending about $800 million in psychiatric drugs in the United States as a whole when Prozac came to market in 1987. We're now spending about $40 billion a year, a fifty-fold increase. So from a business point of view, that's an extraordinary success.

The other problem we've had is that the pharmaceutical companies gave a lot of money to the American Psychiatric Association for various things, starting in 1980. At that time, they began hiring psychiatrists at academic medical schools to serve as consultants, speakers, and advisors. Once they do that, those speakers, who have such legitimacy in our society, are not going to be telling us much about adverse effects or worries about long-term chronicity—they're just going to be celebrating the merits of these drugs. There's a guild interest behind that as well— of course the American Psychiatric Association [APA] has to defend its product. So we see these various monetary interests corrupting the story told to the public: the interests of the pharmaceutical industry, of money going to psychiatrists and to the APA, and the APA's own guild interests. That monetary interest corrupts the story they tell to the public.

Their story is that these drugs are a great help and a great necessity. Yet what is happening in our society as we use these drugs more? We're seeing the burden of mental illness go up, both among adults and as we diagnose more of our kids. We're seeing all the measures of mental health in kids getting worse. And the number of people on disability due to mental illness is soaring in the United States. So when we look at the big picture, this modern paradigm of care where we use these drugs so commonly—is it helping our society reduce the burden of mental illness? Not at all. It's going in the exact opposite direction.

Lobotomy Nation

RLM: One thing this trend is accomplishing is making people docile, isn't it? And that's what you said was going on originally with the mentally ill. With more people in our country on these various zombie medications, people are becoming docile and easier to control. They don't agitate. They don't speak up for themselves. And eventually they don't get represented. What you're talking about here, using the mentally ill as an example, is a movement for an entire culture in the direction of docility, which sounds very dangerous.

RW: It's quite clear that one of the reasons for diagnosing attention-deficit hyperactivity disorder [ADHD] is for prescribing medications that are meant to quiet children and reduce their social interactions. As far as the SSRIs, a lot of people find that they don't feel depressed—they feel numbed out. They just don't care as much as they used to.

RLM: That's what I mean when I say "zombielike."

RW: You hear many people after they've been on these drugs say they don't care so much about their spouse, their kids, their job—they say they can't really get interested in a rainbow—that sort of thing. Sexual dysfunction is much more common than people realize with SSRI usage as well.

RLM: Yeah, that's one of the unspoken aspects of the SSRIs. What I find most painful as a clinician is thinking about what my patients and patients around the country are supposed to do when they hear what you have to say. They're taking these medicines. They've been taking them for a long time. They think they are doing good. They now hear that they may be creating damage. But they also know that if they come off the medicine, the very withdrawal is going to cause them a lot of difficulty—no different than coming off heroin or cocaine; you're going to have a withdrawal effect. They're asking me, "Do I stop taking them? Do I continue taking them? They may be doing the damage, but to stop taking them I have to go through the withdrawal." What a painful position to be in. Well, this is sort of gloomy in a way, folks.

There is one thing that we do know—that's noninvasive and that has been proven to be effective—and it's the least expensive thing possible: that is . . . exercise. Everything that we know about exercise indicates that it may not be a cure, but it certainly alleviates depression and it certainly puts people in a better mood. This is a plea for the use of exercise as your form of treatment, even walking. Robert, thank you for the research you've done, which is so important for my profession and the country at large.

RW: Thank you.

•••

Living Naturally with Julie Holland

Julie Holland is a psychopharmacologist, psychiatrist, and author who has written books on MDMA, marijuana, and pharmaceuticals. In her *New York Times* best-selling book *Moody Bitches,* she reveals the interaction between birth control pills and SSRIs, which cause millions of American women to suffer wide mood swings.

Resisting the "New Normal" of Overmedication
Julie Holland, MD
June 16, 2015

JULIE HOLLAND, MD, is the editor of *Ecstasy: The Complete Guide* (2001) and *The Pot Book* (2010). She also wrote a best seller about her experiences at Bellevue Hospital in New York called *Weekends at Bellevue: Nine Years on the Night Shift at the Psych ER* (2010). Her latest book is *Moody Bitches: The Truth About the Drugs You're Taking, The Sleep You're Missing, The Sex You're Not Having, and What's Really Making You Crazy* (2015).

How a Society on Drugs
Can Return to Living Naturally
The New Normal

RLM: What led you to write the book *Moody Bitches*?

Julie Holland, MD (JH): Twenty years ago, I was practicing psychiatry and a woman came to my office who was really sick and didn't know what was going on. I had to hold her hand and destigmatize the process of taking psychiatric medications, which she really needed. Ten to fifteen years down the road I had people coming to me who didn't have very significant symptoms and basically just wanted to know which medicine they should be on, because they had seen ads for all of these different antidepressants. Their friends were on one thing, their Pilates instructor was on something else, and they were getting a lot of information and advice about which medicine they should take without really looking at whether they were genuinely sick or whether their environment, and their *response* to their environment, was sick.

Sometimes it is the way we are living our lives that is making us feel terrible, and the answer is not to sweep the dirt under the carpet and mask the symptoms by taking something that makes you feel good but to change the way that you're living your life—to take that carpet and beat the heck out of it and sweep your whole floor.

I started seeing this "new normal" where more women were getting on psychiatric medications and antidepressants and antianxiety meds. Then antipsychotics started being used for depression, and I started seeing Big Pharma advertising more to women. They've always targeted women, but it seemed like it was getting worse. I felt like I had to say something. I felt like I needed to turn the ship around. It's a big ship, so it's not going to go quickly, but I felt like I needed to join the parade or lead the parade against everybody being medicated. Being *overly* medicated results in people being unaware of themselves and their environment. They become oblivious to how they're living and how their world is changing.

Natural Movement for Natural Moods

RLM: What's the biggest take-away for a woman who reads this book?

JH: It's the idea of natural moods. Women are naturally cyclical and dynamic. If you're not taking oral contraceptives or antidepressants, it's natural to have times in the month where you feel great and normal at times in the month to feel lousy. The further away we get from nature, the sicker we're going to get. The book is really about returning to nature. I mean, literally going outside and getting some sun. Move your body and get in your body. All of us are spending a lot of time sitting. We're on our phones or computers or in our cars. Just moving your body and being outside with the grass and trees will make you feel better, and you don't necessarily need to keep taking pills every day and living in a way that's very unnatural for you.

RLM: There actually is some scientific evidence now indicating that being out in nature is in and of itself healing. And I know that there are people who are now experimenting with actually lying on the ground, right? What is this about?

JH: It is something called "grounding," and I talk quite a bit about this. This is an evidence-based book. There are about forty pages of notes and hundreds and hundreds of citations. I go into the research behind why exercise is good for you and how being in nature and in sunlight is good for you.

Medicating and Suppressing Natural Moods

JH: Being naturally cyclical, or moody, is really one of women's biggest assets. We have this intuition, empathy, and emotional expression, and we can read other people's emotions. If you mute this sensitivity, you miss out on a lot of information.

RLM: You're implying that there are times of the month when women naturally feel lousy. It's to be expected. So if you feel lousy at certain times of the month, and you track it with your menstrual cycle, then that's just how it is?

JH: Yes.

RLM: That's pretty scary, Julie, because we've got women—fortunately, I think we both agree—going into very high levels of government including the possibility of president. Are we to expect that on a monthly basis they're going to be in a lousy mood, and we'll have to watch out for that? I mean, I don't know if we want that . . .

JH: There are some women who don't have premenstrual syndrome at all, and there are other women who are completely incapacitated by it and require hormones. The majority of other women have some change in their mood over the course of their fertility cycle. That is normal, and there are real advantages to that. But in general, women are quicker to calm themselves and get out of an emotional situation than men are. If you're worried about people being emotional as politicians, I think that's already been covered by men.

RLM: No, I'm not worried about them being emotional. My concern is more that they won't be allowed to be emotional because we live in a culture that wants to somewhat suppress emotion. Remember when George Bach wrote the book *Creative Aggression*—he was saying that some level of very safe fighting is healthy because otherwise, you suppress all this stuff, and you end up full of junk inside.

JH: We all know that if you suppress a behavior, it's going to come out in perverted ways. This idea that you can be celibate or that you can go against your real sexual orientation—it's going to come out in weird ways. For centuries men have had their natural emotional side suppressed. Little boys are taught not to cry—not to act like girls. Women are now getting the message that it's not okay to be emotional, and it's not okay to express or feel your emotions. These are really dangerous, unhelpful, and unhealthful messages. They're getting it also from Big Pharma. The pharmaceutical industry is targeting women in their advertising in women's magazines and daytime talk shows, much more than they are in male-oriented shows. Big Pharma, in regard to psych medications, is exploiting women who feel vulnerable about the fact that they *do* get emotional. I'm not talking about people with major depression who can't get out of bed and their sleep, appetite, and energy levels are completely distorted. They need a psychiatrist and medication. I'm talking about the sort of cosmetic psychopharmacology where more and more women are on psych meds prescribed by nonpsychiatrists, and then they have trouble getting off these meds. It's very difficult to get off antidepressants.

The Drug-Dependence Epidemic

The Importance of Controlled Withdrawal

JH: It's hard to get off antianxiety medicines. It's hard to get off sleeping pills. It's hard to get off stimulants. There are millions of Americans who are taking medicine year after year because they can't stop what they started. They may not need it anymore—their lives may have changed—but they are tolerant and dependent and cannot get off their medicines easily. As soon as they start to pull back on the meds and feel lousy, they become convinced that they have a chemical imbalance and they need to stay on the meds, when really they're experiencing withdrawal.

RLM: That's exactly what Robert Whitaker said on this program and in his book *Anatomy of an Epidemic*—namely, that when people try to get off these medications, then they're running into neurochemical imbalances and thus think they must have needed the medicine to begin with. They think they had better get back on the "needed" medicines but in fact they are going through withdrawal.

JH: Right. There are some psych meds that are harder to get off than others. I've certainly had people say to me, "I've been trying to get off this medicine, but I've been on it an extra ten or twelve years now because I couldn't get off."

I'm good at helping people get off their medicines. It's a slow process, and you need to put a lot of other things in place before you start to pull off these medicines. Sometimes it's not just behavioral changes. Sometimes you need other medicines to make it easier to get off certain other ones.

Worse than Heroin Withdrawal

RLM: When I was practicing chemical dependence treatment full-time, back in the '80s, I was able to detox people from cocaine and heroin in relatively short periods of time. Both drugs are out of your system within three or four days—people can get over withdrawal fairly easily with proper care. Is that not the case with some of the medicines you're talking about? Or should we be creating social model detoxification centers, where people can go away for a week and get these prescription meds out of their system?

JH: People need to understand that coming off psych meds takes weeks or months. It is not in any case just three or four days. It is easier to come off of heroin or cocaine than it is to come off of most prescription psychiatric medications.

RLM: To repeat, here is Dr. Julie Holland is saying that it's easier, in her experience, to come off of cocaine and heroin—which is a lot of my work—than it is to come off the psychiatric medicines that she is encountering. Why is this?

JH: Well, when you take an antidepressant every day, there's all this rebalancing that has to happen with the receptors. When you stop taking the medicine, your brain has to create new receptors and a new balance, and it takes weeks and months. It's a long process and it's very uncomfortable. I often need to use other psychiatric medications to get people off what they're dependent on.

Leveled Emotions on Combination of Contraceptive and Antidepressant

JH: The other thing to mention is that a lot of women are taking oral contraceptives and antidepressants together. And estrogen and serotonin are really linked—yoked to some degree. So when you have naturally high estrogen levels due to the oral contraceptive and high serotonin levels from the antidepressant, and you put those two together, you get a double whammy. It puts you in this hyper-rational, hyper-accommodating state, where you put up with a lot of crap that you normally wouldn't. One advantage of a woman having premenstrual syndrome for a couple of days is that she becomes more critical and more irritated by things. It's a chance to make changes in her environment and potentially in the behavior of people around her.

I had a patient call me from work because she wanted to go up on her antidepressants, because she was crying at work—and you can't cry at work. But when I talked to her about why she was crying, it was because her boss had betrayed and humiliated her in front of her staff, and if she was medicated she wouldn't be so upset about this. So the antidepressants are enabling malignant behavior to go on around her. And it's also not doing her boss any favors or her coworkers any favors.

RLM: I remember when Prozac first came out, Julie. I read an article in the paper by a very astute journalist who said that he was taking Prozac, and it was putting him in a better mood. He was happier. And then he went to his mother's funeral and realized he had no feelings whatsoever, and he said to himself, "This is the price I'm paying for taking this." That's what you're talking about, isn't it?

JH: One of the prices you're paying is that it's going to be very hard to cry and to really feel emotionally connected with people.

RLM: Well, if it's hard to cry, how do you orgasm?

JH: It's nearly impossible for most women on a solid dose of SSRIs to climax. It's a huge, huge problem. In my patient population, women complain about low libido and inability to orgasm, and it is directly affected by the antidepressants they're on.

Tired Soldiers in the Long Battle with Psychiatric Illness
One in Four Women on Psychiatric Medications

RLM: You're saying 25 percent of the adult women in the United States are on psychiatric medications. Is that correct?

JH: In certain demographics it's higher. Now the big thing is antipsychotics. More and more doctors, and not psychiatrists, are prescribing antipsychotics for this kind of malaise and depression that women are experiencing.

RLM: You mean like Abilify [aripiprazole]?

JH: Like Abilify. Abilify was the biggest moneymaker in 2013.

Offering a Quick Fix with No Questions Asked

RLM: How do you feel as a psychiatrist about general practitioners prescribing psychiatric medicine? I know you don't want to criticize your professional colleagues, but that's a fair question.

JH: I don't want to criticize my colleagues, but the truth is that because of the way medicine is set up in America right now, it's all about customers, and getting people in and out of the door, and seeing people for six to ten minutes.

A psychiatrist will spend sixty minutes—maybe even ninety minutes—before they figure out what the diagnosis is and what meds they want to start. A general practitioner or family-practice person will spend six to ten minutes maximum before writing the prescriptions. What should happen is that a psychiatrist should look at the psychiatric history of the family and at genetics and what the treatment response will be before making the decision to start meds. And the biggest thing that no one is talking about is that if you start on meds you are going to feel good, but it's going to be hard to come off.

RLM: What's the exit strategy? If you start these medications, how are you going to get off them? Julie, I want to ask you: Should we be warning people who are taking the psychiatric medicines—who are not under the care of a psychiatrist—who are just getting them from a general practitioner or an internist who sees them for five or six minutes? Should we be giving them some kind of warning? Should we be telling them that they really ought to get to a psychopharmacologist or a psychiatrist? What's the proper thing to do here to protect our citizens?

JH: I think it's always better if you can work with a specialist.

Abilify

RLM: Abilify is an antipsychotic. Zoloft isn't. And Abilify is a major seller in this country. Talk a little about Zoloft and Abilify please.

JH: Well, first of all, Abilify is a really good medicine. It was originally designed to treat schizophrenia, and if you have schizophrenia, it is one of the best antipsychotics you can take. I think it does really amazing things for schizophrenia, and it has worked wonders in my private practice the few times that I did work with schizophrenics. But schizophrenics are only 1 percent of the world's population. If you can target half the world's population, you're going to make a bit more money. So they started targeting women with depression—women who are on meds who weren't getting a really good response from their meds were given Abilify as an add-on to treat depression. They got an FDA indication* [for Abilify] to be used as an add-on and that's really when the money started rolling in for them.

Zoloft

RLM: I want to switch over now and hear you talk about Zoloft.

JH: Zoloft [sertraline] is the most popular antidepressant prescribed among nonpsychiatrists. The way Zoloft got its foothold is that Pfizer would send the drug reps out to family-practice doctors and internists and general practitioners as medicine they could use for patients who were complaining that they were anxious or depressed or having trouble sleeping. The SSRI that I prescribe, that I actually like, is Lexapro. That is the one more commonly prescribed by psychiatrists. However, in 2010, Zoloft sold more units off the shelf than Tide detergent. It's a commonly prescribed and commonly taken drug, but I'm not crazy about it because I believe it has a lot of gastrointestinal side effects. We know it can make people nauseous. It can cause diarrhea—that sort of thing. My big complaint with Zoloft is that it can really make your entire pelvis numb—much less sexually responsive—and make it much more difficult to climax.

---

*A particular use for a medication.

Zoloft vs. Exercise
The Duke Study Revisited

RLM: There was a Duke study comparing Zoloft with exercise, and I will give a brief summary of it. There were three groups in this study. One group received Zoloft, one group received exercise, and one group was given Zoloft and exercise. Remember that SSRIs mean that the little receivers inside the junction box that pull in the Zoloft and distribute it get blocked by this medicine so that serotonin builds up. One group got the Zoloft, one exercise, and one group got both. The people on the exercise did the best. The people on just Zoloft did second best, and the Zoloft-with-exercise group did the worst. What they saw was that the Zoloft actually counters the effect of the exercise. They did a follow-up on that three or four years after and found the same thing, and yet we continue to give Zoloft—I guess in part, Julie, because it seems you can't get some people to exercise. What's the rationale for continuing in the face of this kind of evidence?

JH: I always joke in my office, "If I could just write a prescription for exercise, and you would actually follow it, I would do that." I have actually written down on a piece of prescription paper specific cardio: "Monday, Wednesday, Friday" or "Tuesday, Thursday, Saturday—for forty minutes" to make it more official. It's so much easier to go home and fill prescriptions and take the pills every day than to go outside for a walk, or run, or to get to the gym. I understand it's challenging, and that's why I spend time talking about it and enabling them and figuring out how to make it work for them.

A Universal Prescription for Stress
The Benefits of Exercise and Reducing Inflammation

Runners High: Endocannabinoid and Endorphins

JH: I'll tell patients to get off the subway before their stop so they can walk. I also like my patients doing things like yoga. I went through a long phase of really enjoying running. I think it's important just to find something you don't resent. Optimally, it is something you actually enjoy that makes you feel good. I talk quite a bit in *Moody Bitches* about the cannabinoid system and how cannabis is an anti-inflammatory medicine. I also talk about how the endocannabinoid system floods your brain with cannabinoids when you're doing moderate exercise. There's a lot more research to suggest that the runner's high is not endorphin based but is actually cannabinoid based.

My point is that exercise makes you feel good. It not only has anti-inflammatory properties, but it also helps to grow brain cells. Granted, antidepressants can help to grow brain cells, but you're better off doing it with exercise. This idea that combining antidepressants and exercise will make you feel even worse than antidepressants alone is hard for me to accept, but it makes me more committed to using exercise as a way to help my patients get off their medicine, which is what I do. There are a few things that reliably make it easier for patients to get off their medicine. One of those things is cardiovascular exercise. If I turn someone into a runner, it's much easier for them to taper their meds.

RLM: That's very important. If you're a runner, or let's say an exerciser, Julie Holland is saying it's easier to get off psychiatric medications.

The Two-Way Street of Stress and Inflammation

JH: There are a lot of things that you can do to feel better that don't involve pills. I focus quite a bit on inflammation. Inflammation is the breeding ground for a lot of medical illnesses like arthritis, heart disease, cancer, diabetes, and Alzheimer's. All the autoimmune diseases have a basis in inflammation. It turns out that depression, anxiety, and insomnia also have a basis in inflammation. Much of the advice in my book is really about an anti-inflammatory regimen—things that you can do to decrease chronic inflammation that will help your mood.

RLM: What about the reverse? What about the possibility that anxiety in and of itself is an irritant causing inflammation?

JH: That's a good question, because we know that stress causes inflammation. Yes, it is a two-way street. Anything you can do to decrease stress is going to help to decrease inflammation. And anything you can do to decrease inflammation is going to help you with your mood, with your cognitive functioning, and with your sleep.

FDA Approval by 2021?

Is 2016 the Year of "Coming Out" for Past Psychedelic Users?

More than two years after MAPS founder Rick Doblin, PhD, first joined me on the program, he came back again to talk about progress in his organization's mission to make MDMA the first FDA-approved psychedelic medicine in a therapeutic context.

An Optimistic Forecast

Rick Doblin, PhD

August 18, 2015

RLM: Thirty years ago, Rick Doblin told me he was going to get his PhD and then start a pharmaceutical company. He was going to dedicate his life to working on the legalization of medicines that have been heretofore illegal. He founded MAPS—the Multidisciplinary Association for Psychedelic Studies—a historic pharmaceutical company. Welcome, Rick.

Rick Doblin, PhD (RD): Richard, it's great to be here, and thank you for such an introduction. I don't want to think of myself as historic yet

RLM: Perhaps you're too young to be historic.

RD: I think getting MDMA-assisted psychotherapy approved as a prescription medicine by the FDA and European Medicines Agency will be historic. We are currently anticipating that will happen in 2021, so I've got an awful lot of work before the word "historic" would really qualify.

RLM: Some of us look at you that way already, Rick, because the work MAPS has done around the globe has been a breath of fresh air for those of us in the professions of psychology and psychiatry. Those of us who were around when MDMA was legal and saw the benefits to ourselves and to our patients look at what you're doing as historic because there's light at the end of what has been a very long tunnel of government suppression of information.

A Thirtieth Anniversary Celebration

RLM: As you recently said publicly at your wonderful lecture at the old Federal Reserve building in San Francisco, when introducing Stan Grof, we're looking at having MDMA as a legally prescribed medicine in the year 2021. The whole audience stood and applauded because all these professions are waiting for this event. And that's, I think, what makes it historic.

RD: Our thirtieth anniversary is 2016. I started MAPS one year after MDMA was criminalized in 1985. We were thinking of having an event in the Bay Area, where we'd follow the lead of the gay rights movement. What they achieved was largely because people came out and said they were gay. Instead of hiding in the shadows, people acknowledged who they were. We're looking to possibly do a similar event of people with mainstream credibility, but who have been quiet about the influence of LSD on their lives. Maybe if a bunch of people were to do it together it might be less worrisome. We're thinking about it as a big coming out as far as psychedelics' influence on people's lives.

RLM: I think that's an excellent idea. I feel strongly that an extremely high percentage of the psychologists and psychiatrists that I know who experienced MDMA when it was legal, in their therapist's office, will come out for what you're talking about and go public.

RD: That's fantastic.

Signs of Hope at the
American Psychiatric Association

RD: I actually got the idea at the American Psychiatric Association annual conference this year in May in Toronto. About twelve thousand psychiatrists from around the world come to it. For the first year in many years MAPS and the Heffter Research Institute were able to get a three-hour seminar on psychedelic-assisted psychotherapy. Also, MAPS purchased a table in the exhibit hall where Big Pharma had all their tables—but they didn't have *tables*. *We* had a $5,000 table, which was just a table. *They* had massive exhibits that cost hundreds of thousands of dollars. So we kind of felt like we had arrived with this seminar and our little table.

But what we didn't predict was fantastic. The president of the American Psychiatric Association is president for just one year, and the last thing they do is preside over the conference that they have organized during the prior year. The president put an interview that he did with Ram Dass [Richard Alpert] on the schedule. There was an hour and a half with discussion after this interview. We were shocked to see that Ram Dass was having an honored place at the American Psychiatric Conference—Ram Dass being a psychologist rather than a psychiatrist and being associated with Tim Leary and Ralph Metzner at Harvard for psychedelic research.

During the interview, the president—the sitting president of the

APA—announced that when he was nineteen years old he took LSD and had a profound spiritual experience. He dropped out of college, traveled around, studied Zen—became kind of an itinerant Zen monk—and then eventually he had a dream that told him to become a psychiatrist. He was basically saying that LSD was responsible for him becoming a psychiatrist, and he had kept this quiet. This was at sixty-five years old and at the pinnacle of his career, he felt safe enough to acknowledge the role of LSD in his life.

RLM: And that is why I think you're going to get tremendous support from psychologists and psychiatrists in going public, because there are so many of us who are in our late sixties and seventies, like myself, who are old enough to have been administered these medicines while they were still legal. There are enough of us around who took LSD when it was legal. I took MDMA for the first time in the office of my therapist—Robert Kantor, who started the Pacific Graduate School of Psychology. He regularly used it with me while it was legal.

All of us who have taken it are experientially aware of the profound positive effects that these medicines had on us and our patients. We've been waiting in the wings for decades for you to come along—and it happens to be you.

Setting Modern Psychiatry Straight
A New Model for Psychotherapy

RLM: We have to return to the legal use of these medicines, because modern psychiatry is adrift—the pharmaceutical companies are creating medicines that Robert Whitaker says are wreaking havoc with neurotransmitters [see chapter 5]. The medicines that are being used are not helpful—they may be making people suffer more, not less. And here we have these other medicines that thousands, if not tens of thousands, of us professionals have experienced to have positive effects.

RD: We believe therapists who want to work with these substances will be more effective if they've tried them themselves. In some ways that's an obvious statement—if you want to study yoga, you go to somebody that practices yoga; or if you want to study meditation you go study with somebody that actually meditates.

It makes intuitive sense that if you want psychedelic-assisted therapy you should ideally go to somebody that has had these experiences. Many younger psychiatrists and psychologists that grew up during this period of the backlash have received very little in the way of education about psychedelics, and the education they have received has been largely negative. They are taught that it causes psychosis—people go crazy—and that we have to deal with them at the hospitals.

From a view of integrating psychedelic-assisted psychotherapy into mainstream psychiatry and psychotherapy, MDMA is more likely to be adopted by mainstream psychiatrists and psychotherapists. We've already seen that to be the case in that we have FDA approval for a protocol. We've been able to bring in therapists from Israel, from the Veterans Administration, from the United States, and from England and give them MDMA experiences in a legal, controlled, and scientific way to help them be more effective when they work on our studies. I think there would have been several of those people that would not have volunteered for psilocybin or LSD but were willing to volunteer for receiving MDMA.

No Such Thing as a One-Dose Miracle Cure

RLM: What are the viewpoints of the professions of clinical psychology and psychiatry regarding the thousands of research studies that were done with LSD while it was legal that indicated profound benefits, particularly the research out of England on treating alcoholism?

RD: The consensus is that there were some remarkable recoveries but that when you look at the evidence, there were flaws with the meth odological design in light of our modern understanding of randomized placebo-controlled double-blind studies. The follow-ups were showing that the benefits lasted six months, but they didn't persist beyond that. The treatment model used back then was what I would characterize as a "one-dose miracle cure." They tested whether you could give patients one overwhelming experience of LSD to try to produce a spiritual experience, bringing up from people's unconscious, into awareness, what they were suppressing. This was supposed to help them see the consequences of what they were doing and then help them have this unitive, mystical, connective experience that they could draw strength from. This method could be insufficient without aftercare programs to help people start a new life and refrain from alcoholism on a long-term basis.

And while it did work with some people, the whole treatment model was unrealistically idealistic in the sense that it was this one-dose model. What we understand now is that to really change deep-seated patterns of addiction, personality patterns, pains, depressions, or anxiety, it usually takes more than one session and it takes a lot more focus on the integration process. When people look back at the evidence from prior studies, the results tend to get dismissed as being a psychedelic afterglow that fades over time.

Challenging the Annuity Model

RLM: I'm thinking now of Roland Griffiths, who was on this program. I know in his study they gave psilocybin once, and subjects have had positive results a year later.

If one dose can, on average, help people for six months, that's phenomenal. When you compare that to the SSRIs and the various medicines that Big Pharma is giving us—where you have to take the medicine every single day for the rest of your life, thereby paying an annuity—to be able to take a medicine once and get a six-month result is truly phenomenal.

RD: Yeah—those were mostly healthy people looking for spiritual experiences, and they did work with cancer patients with anxiety. The research from the past suggests several things. It suggests that LSD and the classic psychedelics can be given safely. It is also preliminary evidence of efficacy sustained over a relatively short period of time and that with a more rigorous methodological design of the studies, and with greater focus on the integration process, these substances could be a remarkable new addition to psychiatry.

Instead of practicing psychiatry, many psychiatrists don't even study psychotherapy at all and are agents of the pharmaceutical industry. They prescribe medications in fifteen-minute appointments with their patients. They don't really understand psychotherapy. We've also seen that psychoanalysis has had a lot of assumptions that are not scientifically verified, and the "talking cure" only goes so deep for a lot of people. That model has fallen into disrepute among psychiatrists and has left them unprepared for psychedelic-assisted psychotherapy, because they really have to hone their skills in the psychotherapeutic process. So what we're basically trying to do is introduce a new model that some psychiatrists and psychotherapists will be willing to do. It's more labor intensive in the short run, but it has the benefits of easing suffering and costing less money in the long run.

Breaking through to Phase III Approval

RD: We will be completing our international series of Phase II pilot studies at the end of 2015, and we will have the primary outcome data from around 105 PTSD patients. We will be able to show that in our experimental conditions that are carefully controlled, with pure MDMA—with lots of preparation and integration, a male-female co-therapist team working with people for the full eight hours, and the whole time of their integration and preparation sessions—*under those circumstances* we're able to deliver MDMA psychotherapy without any lasting negative side effects and with remarkable evidence of efficacy.

The evidence is so remarkable, in fact, that we considered applying to the FDA for what is so-called "breakthrough therapy designation." This is a program to accelerate the development of drugs for serious and life-threatening illnesses for which there's a large group of patients for whom other available treatments have not worked. Usually it's for new cancer drugs that have a genetic basis for certain kinds of people with certain genetic histories, and that's the way in which the FDA can accelerate that. There's only been one drug for mental illness—for psychiatric purposes—that's been approved under breakthrough therapy, and it was esketamine, an isomer of ketamine for suicidal refractory depression. So we think we've got about a fifty-fifty chance of getting this designation. However, after a meeting with our FDA consultant, we decided that it would be best to just go forward with a standard FDA End of Phase II meeting,* since the remarkable results and high-profile nature of MDMA meant that our application to the FDA would still receive attention and guidance of senior management, and the designs of our Phase II studies weren't exactly the kind that the FDA wanted to see for breakthrough therapy designation. We decided to take the standard approach.

The End of Phase II meeting is a good way to present the information to the FDA as part of the negotiations for Phase III, which is the studies that count to make a drug into a medicine—the large-scale, multisite, randomized placebo-controlled studies.

We're anticipating starting those around early 2017. We will be completing them and hopefully getting approval by around 2021. We currently estimate those studies will cost around $22 million. We have raised already about half of the cost in actual money and also have

---

*The purpose of the End of Phase II meeting is to "facilitate interaction between the FDA and sponsors who seek guidance related to clinical trial design . . . for better dose response estimation and dose selection, and other related issues." From U.S. Department of Health and Human Services, Federal Drug Administration, Center for Drug Evaluation and Research, "Guidance for Industry: End of Phase 2A Meetings," September 2009, 4; www.fda.gov/downloads/Drugs/. . . /Guidances/ucm079690.pdf (accessed June 5, 2017).

pledges. We recently got $5 million pledged—a million a year for five years—from Dr. Bronner's Magic Soaps.

•••

There was a time, in recent history, when the people of the world believed the planet was flat; a handful of scientists were demonized for their belief that the world was round. Pythagoras is often credited for establishing the world as round.

There was a time, in recent history, when people believed that the earth revolved around the sun. Then came Galileo.

There was time, quite recently, when people believed that thunder was an expression of God's anger and lightning bolts were thrown at us by God himself. Then came Benjamin Franklin.

There was a brief period in history, lasting about two thousand years, when people believed that sex was bad and dirty. Then came Kinsey.

We are living in a time when government leaders are still making policies based on self-interest, materialism, morality, ideology, and religion. To advance their irrational beliefs these misguided leaders have been waging a war that has extended to science itself and has cost the lives of patients—denied access to certain medicines called psychedelic—as well as untold numbers of people who have been criminalized for nothing more than ingesting something they were denied access to. We will look back on this period the same way we look back on the period when the world was thought to be flat.

During this present historic period of suppression of science, a small group of scientists around the world persevered in the face of career-consuming obstacles and have brought us life-changing information. It is our good fortune that these scientists have taken the time to sit for the interviews presented in this book and have spoken to us in language readily understandable. The data collected by these scientists clearly informs us that the medicines classified as psychedelic have huge potential both as a healing modality, perhaps only limited by our own creativity in using them, and also as an instrument for consciousness expansion. These psychedelic medicines also provide an avenue in the field of epigenetics, whereby we will go inside ourselves and self-sculpt our very genetic inheritance. We are also reminded, by the scientists, as well as our own observations, that the best of medicines can become a dangerous drug when taken improperly.

As we were editing this book, three thousand people from around the world—many of whom are scientists—gathered in Oakland, California, for the Psychedelic Science Conference sponsored by America's MAPS and England's Beckley Foundation. All of the scientists in this book presented one or more papers at the conference.

Information can be suppressed ad nauseam but not ad infinitum.

•••

To support research into the therapeutic uses of psychedelic medicines, consider making a donation to MAPS, the Multidisciplinary Association for Psychedelic Studies, a 501(c)(3) nonprofit research and educational organization that develops medical, legal, and cultural contexts for people to benefit from the careful uses of psychedelics and marijuana.

Acknowledgments

Between age fifty-five and seventy-five I studied government with particular emphasis on American history 1743–1812. It was during this period that I came to see myself as a proud member of the American Revolution. In my heart I was with Franklin when he was humiliated before the court of King George. I sat proudly with Jefferson when he Franklin, and Adams wrote the Declaration of Independence. I stood tall with the signers of the Declaration, in Philadelphia, and I clearly remember the smell of the butcher across the street. I rowed with Washington when he crossed the Delaware and attacked the German mercenaries hired by King George to kill us. I marched with Hamilton when he organized a regiment in Manhattan. I burned the midnight oil with Hamilton when he wrote the Federalist papers, and again with Madison when he wrote our Constitution.

I am eternally grateful to our Founding Fathers for leading us out submission to the king and into being citizens equal under the law. My heart sings appreciation for how they led us out of religious influence on government and into the separation of church and state.

As a patriotic American I am deeply saddened that for the last fifty years our government has not had the wisdom to proactively support to the utmost, scientific research into psychedelic medicine. Psychedelic medicines have the most potential for unlocking the innermost workings of our consciousness and directing the epigenetic expression of the building blocks of our material being: deoxyribonucleic acid (DNA).

As a patriotic American I am also saddened that our government has yet to realize the right of Americans to ingest anything they choose, in the privacy of their homes, so long as they do not do harm to any another human being who may be in their home. To deny this right turns honest citizens into breakers of the law but never prevents massive experimentation.

I wish to thank the following people for their work and their collaborative efforts in making *Psychedelic Medicine* possible; they have made a significant contribution to us all. First, we are indebted to the scientists whose work is documented in this book. Their perseverance in the face of challenges and obstacles, as well as potential threats to their careers, has provided our world with important scientific information having monumental potential for healing and creativity. It has been my distinct privilege to interview each of them.

I thank my friend Mike Dell'Ara, who played a key role in the creation of this volume. Mike has served as my trusted confidante and dedicated radio engineer. His clarity of friendship is inspiring. My friend Charlie Diest is the sina qua non of this book. He built a website, Psychepedia.org, that contains the interviews in this book. He supervised the transcription of the interviews and much more. Mike and Charlie, thank you!

I also thank my editor, Jennie Marx, and the staff of Inner Traditions/Bear & Co. They provided essential support.

Index

BOOKS OF RELATED INTEREST

Psychedelic Healing
The Promise of Entheogens for Psychotherapy and Spiritual Development
by Neal M. Goldsmith, Ph.D.

The Psychedelic Explorer's Guide
Safe, Therapeutic, and Sacred Journeys
by James Fadiman, Ph.D.

DMT: The Spirit Molecule
A Doctor's Revolutionary Research into the Biology of Near-Death
and Mystical Experiences
by Rick Strassman, M.D.

Psychedelic Consciousness
Plant Intelligence for Healing Ourselves and Our Fragmented World
by Daniel Grauer

Psychedelics and Spirituality
The Sacred Use of LSD, Psilocybin, and MDMA
for Human Transformation
Edited by Thomas B. Roberts, Ph.D.

Cannabis and Spirituality
An Explorer's Guide to an Ancient Plant Spirit Ally
Edited by Stephen Gray

Visionary Ayahuasca
A Manual for Therapeutic and Spiritual Journeys
by Jan Kounen

The Ayahuasca Experience
A Sourcebook on the Sacred Vine of Spirits
Edited by Ralph Metzner, Ph.D.

Inner Traditions • Bear & Company
P.O. Box 388
Rochester, VT 05767
1-800-246-8648
www.InnerTraditions.com

Or contact your local bookseller